The Pocket Guide to Critical Appraisal

The Pocket Guide to Critical Appraisal

SECOND EDITION

Iain K. Crombie

University of Dundee
Dundee, UK

WILEY Blackwell

Registered Offices
John Wiley & Sons, Inc., 111 River Street, Hoboken, NJ 07030, USA
John Wiley & Sons Ltd, The Atrium, Southern Gate, Chichester, West Sussex, PO19 8SQ, UK

Editorial Office
9600 Garsington Road, Oxford, OX4 2DQ, UK

For details of our global editorial offices, customer services, and more information about Wiley products visit us at www.wiley.com.

Library of Congress Cataloging-in-Publication Data Applied for

Paperback ISBN: 9781119835240

Cover Design: Wiley
Cover Image: © Govindanmarudhai/Getty Images

Set in 10.5/13pt STIXTwoText by Straive, Chennai, India

SKY8461C535-F3AD-434F-95E6-80877214C245_052422

Contents

Acknowledgements

I am grateful to the University of Dundee for providing the facilities to research and write the second edition of this book. The success of the first edition was due in no small part to my colleagues for their support and encouragement. As the style and much of the content of this new edition follows the original, I am pleased to be able to thank them again for their help. Special thanks are due to Geraldine Fardon whose constructive comments highlighted imprecise, vague, and confusing text. I take full responsibility for any remaining flaws.

Acknowledgements

Preface to the First Edition

This book was written to meet the needs of health professionals as medicine moves to be evidence-based. The initial idea arose during discussion with younger colleagues and students on difficulties of interpreting the medical literature. It quickly became apparent that their needs would be best met by a short book detailing criteria for critical appraisal.

The book is organised in two parts. The first five chapters provide an introduction to critical appraisal of quantitative research, indicating how papers can be read and how the results can be interpreted. Experienced researchers could easily omit these chapters. The final six chapters provide annotated checklists for critical appraisal. The first of these contains the general questions which can be asked of any study using a quantitative methodology. The succeeding five chapters review in turn the questions which are specific for each quantitative method. For convenience each of these five chapters concludes with a combined list of general and specific questions.

The book has been written to be simple and quick to use. Technical terms are avoided where possible, and the assessment criteria are explained but not justified. A larger and less accessible text would have been needed to give a proper rationale for each the checklists. To keep this a pocket guide, it was also decided to omit evaluations of other topics such as qualitative methods, health economics, clinical audit, decision analysis, and screening tests. An argument could be made for the inclusion of each, but to include them all would nearly double the size of the book. I hope the checklists prove useful.

Preface to the First Edition

Preface to the Second Edition

Several developments have highlighted the need for a second edition of this book. Recent work, particularly from the new discipline of meta-research, has provided important evidence for critical appraisal. By examining and comparing large numbers of studies, this research has clarified the nature of and impact of many sources of bias. A separate development is the recognition that critical appraisal should distinguish between the risk of bias and the value of the findings to individuals, health care systems, and the wider society. Critical appraisal checklists should provide separate sets of questions for the two issues. Finally, many years of teaching critical appraisal skills have provided the author with an understanding of the difficulties that students and health professionals encounter when evaluating papers. These developments have led to improvements in the guidance given in this book.

This new edition follows the format and the spirit of the first: it is written to be easy to use and, where possible, technical terms are avoided. However, substantial modifications have been made. A new Introduction clarifies the aims of critical appraisal. The second chapter, entitled 'Do Not Read the Paper', is also new; it provides a simple method for eliciting the information needed for critical appraisal from published studies. This is supported by Chapter 5, 'The In-Depth Interrogation', which is a much-amended version of the original 'Standard Appraisal Questions'. In addition, Chapter 4 on 'Interpreting the Results' has been updated in line with current views on the nature of statistical significance and the interpretation of confidence intervals.

All of the chapters that provide checklists for critical appraisal of specific research designs have been revised and updated, particularly Chapter 9, 'Appraising Randomised Controlled Trials', and Chapter 11, 'Appraising Systematic Reviews'. A new chapter for the critical appraisal of cohort studies that evaluate interventions has been added. This research design is now being frequently used in medical research (the separate chapter on conventional cohort studies has been retained). All the checklists distinguish between critical and important sources of bias and they evaluate risk of bias separately from value.

Two new chapters at the end of the book provide methods for synthesising the findings of critical appraisal. One provides a method for summarising risk of bias. The second explores the important concept of certainty of evidence and describes how it is assessed. A further new chapter reviews the wide range of factors that determine the value of research findings to society as a whole. This second edition provides a much-needed update to the guidance on critical appraisal.

CHAPTER 1

Introduction to Critical Appraisal

Critical appraisal is the process of assessing the strengths and weaknesses of published studies. It involves a structured and rigorous evaluation of all the stages of the research, from design to analysis and interpretation. All studies have imperfections, so the question is not if there are flaws, but whether they are likely to be important. Critical appraisal is a method of systematically examining research studies to determine the worth of their findings.

The aims of critical appraisal

Critical appraisal assesses two issues: bias in study design or conduct, and the value that the findings have for clinical practice. Bias occurs when systematic errors distort the results of a study. For example, a clinical trial should provide a good estimate of the benefit of a treatment, but weaknesses in design or conduct could produce a misleading estimate. There are many types of bias and

The Pocket Guide to Critical Appraisal, Second Edition. Iain K. Crombie.
© 2022 John Wiley & Sons Ltd. Published 2022 by John Wiley & Sons Ltd.

these are explored through a series of questions that examine the main deficiencies in research.

The value of findings is the extent to which they will provide benefits for patients or the general population. Many factors contribute to the value of research findings. For a clinical trial, this would include the size of the treatment benefit, the importance of the outcome measure to patients, and whether the patients to be treated in a clinical setting are similar to the participants in the study. As with bias, there are sets of questions that assess value.

Three stages of critical appraisal

The critical appraisal of a paper is conducted in three stages: identify the research design, select the appropriate appraisal tool for that study, and apply the tool to assess the bias and the value of the research. This section introduces these stages, with subsequent chapters explaining in detail how to carry them out.

Identify the research design

Research studies can ask different types of questions. Some may be concerned with the effectiveness of treatments; others may investigate the likely prognosis of an illness. The research design should be matched to the research question. To evaluate treatment effectiveness a randomised controlled trial would be used, whereas prognosis would be investigated by a cohort study. The other designs are surveys, case–control studies, cohort studies that test interventions, and systematic reviews. Chapter 3 of this book provides guidance on identifying the correct design.

Select the appropriate appraisal tool

Critical appraisal tools have been developed to enable a forensic evaluation of research studies. They provide lists of questions that probe all aspects of the methods used and the results obtained. Judgements can then be made about the bias and value of the research. This book presents appraisal tools for the six most common research designs in medical research (Chapters 6–11).

A key feature of the questions on bias is that they distinguish between critical and important sources of bias. For each research design there are a few crucial steps which, if conducted poorly, are very likely to lead to misleading findings. Flaws in the other steps are less likely to cause serious bias. Only when several of these flaws occur are serious concerns raised.

Value, the usefulness or worth of a finding to individuals and to society, is more difficult to assess. Assessing the potential for improving health is usually straightforward, but often some pieces of information, such as the importance of the findings to patients, are not available. Decisions about value can use information from several sources and require judgement to balance many complex issues.

Apply the tool to assess the bias and the value of the research

The critical appraisal questions can only be answered by identifying key pieces of information from relevant sections of a paper. Chapter 2 provides a simple method for extracting the key pieces of information from a research paper. Careful reflection on what the questions reveal enables an assessment of the quality of the research study.

The appraisal questions presented in this book are structured to lead to one of three answers: yes, no, or not enough information to decide. Selecting the appropriate option is not a simple tick box process. Critical appraisal involves pausing to think about the implications of each limitation, and whether it could seriously affect the interpretation of the study's findings. Sometimes there will be insufficient information to answer a question. As decisions in medicine affect patients, it is usually better to be cautious in drawing conclusions.

In summary, critical appraisal assesses the bias and the value of research studies. By identifying the research design, the appropriate appraisal tool is selected. It asks probing questions about the design of the study and the way it was conducted, analysed, and interpreted. Chapter 2 describes a simple method for extracting the information from published papers to facilitate critical appraisal.

Do Not Read the Paper

The most important piece of advice when appraising a scientific paper is: do not read the paper. Scientific papers are complicated, information dense, and full of technical jargon – they cannot be read like a newspaper article. They are written for experts and prioritise technical correctness over ease of understanding. The research design is often complex, and the statistical analysis sophisticated. Papers are written with the assumption that the reader is familiar with the scientific terms and the methodologies used. Reading every word from the Introduction to the Discussion may lead to confusion.

A better approach is to interrogate the paper, asking questions to make it reveal the information about study design and conduct. Unlike reading, which is a passive process, critical appraisal searches out the key pieces of information about a study. Interrogation puts the reader in charge, directing questions at different sections of the paper, identifying and checking the information in the paper. This approach provides a quicker appraisal of a paper because it focuses on the important features of research studies. It probes not just what was done, but how well it was done. Sometimes the authors of papers try to gloss over weaknesses in their study. Interrogation will identify flaws that reading may miss. It provides all the information needed to evaluate the risk of bias and value of the results.

The initial interrogation

The initial interrogation involves delving into some sections of the paper to get a feel for what the study is about. The aim is to start constructing a mental map of the study, not to engage in a serious appraisal. The main benefit of the map is that it allows you to slot subsequent pieces of information into a mental framework. This simplifies the task of understanding the paper and helps you organise the information it contains. The process uses four questions.

What does the title reveal about the study?

The interrogation begins with the title. Good titles should indicate the patient group being investigated, the research design used, and why the study is being done. Sometimes titles are written to be catchy rather than informative, but even then, they should provide one or two facts about the study. The title provides the first indication of what the study is about.

Does the abstract help in constructing the mental map?

The Abstract usually gives key information about the four main sections of the paper: the Introduction, Methods, Results, and Discussion. Ideally it will clarify the study aim, the research design that was used, the main findings and their implications. Together with the title, the Abstract should enable you to construct a provisional map of the paper. However, this is not guaranteed. Information in the Abstracts may be presented to impress rather than to be informative. The provisional map should be tested by comparing what it says with the information presented in the Introduction and the Methods sections.

Does the introduction confirm the aims?

The aims of the study are usually presented towards the end of the Introduction. They may be phrased as hypotheses to be tested or as questions to be answered. The absence of a clear statement of aims could mean that the authors had no real idea of what they were trying to find out. Research studies with unclearly stated aims are often of poor quality.

Does the methods section explain how the study aims will be achieved?

The Methods section should explain how all aspects of the study were carried out. The descriptions in this section are often brief and difficult to follow. This section should clarify how participants were recruited, the data that were collected, and the statistical techniques that were used. Often, the research design, which should explain how the study aims will be achieved, is not clearly stated. To assist with this limitation, Chapter 3 provides guidance on identifying the research design. It outlines the main features and the key terms indicative of the six most common research designs.

The in-depth interrogation

The initial interrogation should provide a provisional map of the paper into which information about the sources of bias and the value of the study findings can be fitted. This process requires an in-depth interrogation using detailed questions which probe the quality of the study. These questions are described in Chapters 5–11. Before reading these chapters, it may be helpful to review Chapter 3 'Identifying the Research Design' and Chapter 4 'Interpreting the Results'.

CHAPTER 3

Identifying the Research Design

The first step in critical appraisal is to identify the research design used in a study so the appropriate appraisal checklist can be selected. This chapter provides an outline of the common research designs to aid their identification. It does not provide a full description of each method, but instead gives sufficient detail to confirm which design was used.

Surveys

Surveys are often used to estimate how common something is: how many people have high blood pressure, or how many suffer from chronic pain. They can also investigate associations between factors: is it more common in men or women; does the frequency of high blood pressure vary with age? Surveys can study whole populations; for example, to establish the proportion of people who currently smoke cigarettes. Or they can investigate specific groups;

The Pocket Guide to Critical Appraisal, Second Edition. Iain K. Crombie.
© 2022 John Wiley & Sons Ltd. Published 2022 by John Wiley & Sons Ltd.

for example, they could explore the health beliefs of pregnant women, or the frequency of loneliness in persons aged between 65 and 90 years.

Essential features

Surveys take samples from a target group or population. The idea behind this is that a well-taken sample contains almost as much information as would come from studying the whole population. In principle, surveys obtain a complete list of the group or population of interest from which a sample of individuals is selected for further study. The selection is carried out randomly (not haphazardly), such that each individual has an equal chance of being chosen. In practice, a complete list may not be available and alternative approaches such as cluster sampling can be used (these more complicated designs are not described here). The important points are that selection of individuals uses random sampling and that the sample obtained is representative of a target population.

Complications

Surveys usually do not have a separate control or comparison group, so studies that have them are not surveys. However, in the analysis of surveys one subgroup in the sample may be compared against another (e.g. men versus women, or old versus young). Comparisons are being made, but there is no sense in which one group is acting as a control to another group. All the individuals have been selected at the same time and an internal comparison is made.

Terms of identification

Use of the term *survey* in a paper should identify the method, but sometimes the term is used for what is really a cohort study. *Cross-sectional* is a helpful term because it is seldom used with any other research method. *Prevalence*, the frequency of something in a sample, also suggests that a study is a survey. The terms *sample* and *random sample* are unhelpful because they often appear in the description of the other research designs. The terms *simple*, *cluster*, or *systematic* can be used with the word *sampling* to describe different ways of drawing a sample, e.g. *cluster sampling*. These terms are seldom used with the other research designs. The phrase *stratified sampling* is also used in surveys, but the word *stratified* can also be used in randomised controlled trials (RCTs).

Cohort studies

Cohort studies are used to find out what happens to study participants over time. It is the method of choice for studying disease prognosis, or for investigating the consequences of exposure to potentially harmful agents. For example, studies could investigate how long patients with acute low back pain take to recover, or how many people who smoke subsequently develop lung cancer. Whatever the topic, a group of individuals is identified and followed up to see what events befall them. Most commonly the aim is to determine whether exposure to a potentially noxious substance leads to an increased risk of a disease. Sometimes the interest is in whether potentially beneficial substances, such as dietary vitamins or fish oils, reduce the risk of disease.

Essential features

The defining characteristic of cohort studies is the element of time: in cohort studies time flows forwards. A set of individuals is identified at one point in time and followed up to a later time to ascertain what has happened. These studies are called prospective cohort studies. When studying the impact of some exposure, cohort studies often have a comparison or control group. The controls are usually identified at around the same time and followed for the same length of time. This type of cohort study is called a *concurrent cohort study*.

Many cohort studies do not have a control group; instead they can make internal comparisons. For example, a cohort could recruit a large sample from the general population and identify who smoked and who did not. The whole sample would be followed up for several years to determine whether lung cancer occurs more frequently in smokers than in non-smokers.

Complications

Some cohort studies identify the group from some time in the past and follow them up to the present. These studies might at first appear to be looking backwards in time, but they are not. Historical records are used, and time flows forwards from the point at which the individuals are identified. This type of design is usually called a *retrospective cohort study*. (Note the term *historical cohort study* is used when the exposed group is recruited from one period and the comparison group comes from an earlier period.)

Terms of identification

The terms *prospective* and *longitudinal* suggest a cohort study, although these terms are also used in clinical trials. The term *retrospective* is used for one type of cohort study, but is also used with case–control studies.

Case–control studies

Case–control studies ask what makes a group of individuals different from a control or comparison group. Often the study group will have a disease, which the control group do not have. For example, the cases could be women with breast cancer and the controls could be women of similar age who do not have the disease. The study compares the characteristics of the cases and controls to identify the factors from the past that might have caused the disease. The control group is often selected to be similar to the cases in factors such as age, gender, and life circumstances. This type of study can also explore why some people behave in a particular way. For example, a study could explore why some patients miss clinic appointments, by comparing those who fail to attend with those who do attend.

Essential features

Case–control studies look backwards in time from some event (e.g. the diagnosis of breast cancer or failing to attend a clinic) to try to identify factors in the past that might explain why that event occurred. The direction of time is crucial for distinguishing between cohort studies and case–control studies: cohort studies look forwards; case–control studies backwards.

Complications

The use of a control group is not a defining characteristic, since RCTs always have one, and cohort studies often do.

Terms of identification

Several terms are used for this type of study including: *case–control*, *case–referent*, *case-comparator*, and *case-comparison*. Because the method looks backwards in time it is sometimes called a *retrospective study*, but this term can be used with cohort studies.

RCTs

The RCT should be the easiest method to identify. This design is used to test whether one health care intervention is superior to another. RCTs are most often used to test drugs, but they can be used to investigate many different types of health care interventions: surgery, vaccination, anti-pressure sore mattresses, and health education. RCTs often compare a new treatment against the currently accepted best treatment. If there is no existing treatment, the new one is compared against a placebo (an inert substance or a dummy procedure).

Essential features

RCTs are always concerned with effectiveness. The key element of this design is that patients are randomly allocated to receive a new treatment or to the conventional one (or a placebo). The outcome of the new treatment is compared with that of the conventional one, identifying which is superior. RCTs are also concerned with the side effects of treatments. Most RCTs compare two treatments, but sometimes more than two treatments can be investigated. This adds complexity to the conduct and analysis of the study, although the resulting study is a valid RCT.

Complications

The phrase clinical trial is often used as shorthand for an RCT. However, clinical trial can refer to studies in which patients are allocated treatment in a non-random way (non-randomised studies). For example, cohort studies can be used to assess effectiveness: a group of treated patients and an independent control group are followed up to see which group gains most benefit.

Terms of identification

The term *randomisation* almost always identifies an RCT, as does the equivalent phrase *random allocation*. (Note that the term *random selection* may refer to a survey.) The terms *blinding*, *placebo*, *effectiveness*, *efficacy*, and *evaluation*, or phrases like *assess the value of* or *improve the outcome*, can be used in both RCTs and non-randomised studies.

Cohort studies that evaluate the effectiveness of interventions

An increasingly common research design is a special type of cohort study that evaluates the effectiveness of treatments. It compares the outcomes among a group of patients given one treatment with outcomes in other patients who have the same disease but were given a different treatment. The difference from a conventional RCT is that patients are not randomised to treatments. Instead the clinician responsible for the patient decides which treatment should be given. This type of study evaluates treatments as they are used in routine clinical practice. A common form of this design uses electronic health records to identify patients with a defined disease and the treatments that they were given. The effects of the treatments on the outcome measures are also obtained from electronic data. When the two groups are recruited and followed up in the same time period, this design is called a *concurrent cohort study*. In a different form of this design, recently diagnosed patients are given the new treatment and are compared with patients from the past who were given a different treatment. These studies are called *historical cohort studies*.

Essential features

The essential feature of this design is that the treatment patients receive is selected by the doctors who are responsible for their care, based on an assessment of their specific clinical circumstances. Rather than being randomised to treatment groups, clinical judgement is used to decide which treatment will be best for each patient. As a result, the patients given one treatment may differ systematically from those given the other treatment. This is the major weakness of the research design, as the two groups of patients will be different at the start of the study (i.e. before they receive their treatment).

Complications

A special type of cohort treatment study is the *quasi-randomised study*. In this design patients are assigned by the researchers to treatment groups using a non-random method such as date of clinic appointment (assignment by alternate days) or date of birth (assignment by odd or even dates). Because the assignment process is predictable, it could be tampered with, creating a risk of bias. This design is best viewed as similar to an RCT, but one at high risk of bias due to poor concealment of treatment allocation.

Terms of identification

There are no specific terms which identify this research design. The terms *concurrent cohort study* and *historical cohort study* could refer to this design, but they could also refer to conventional cohort studies (those which do not evaluate the effectiveness of treatments). The term *non-randomised study* is often used for this type of study, although that label refers to a group of research designs which include case–control studies, surveys, interrupted time series, and case series.

Systematic reviews

Systematic reviews seek to identify all the papers published on a specific health topic to obtain a summary of the findings from all the relevant studies. They commonly use the statistical technique of meta-analyses to combine the findings from each study. In effect, meta-analysis produces results which are comparable with those from one very large study. This approach overcomes the weakness of individual studies, which, because of their small size, can be greatly affected by the play of chance.

Essential features

Systematic reviews search electronic databases of research studies, such as MEDLINE, EMBASE, and CINAHL, to locate published studies, using carefully chosen combinations of key terms. Papers are carefully screened to identify the relevant ones. The chosen papers are commonly referred to as the primary studies. Key data items, such as effect size, standard deviation, and sample size, are extracted from each study. These data are usually, but not always, combined to provide an overall estimate of effect size using meta-analysis.

Complications

There are no complications. The design of a systematic review differs substantially from all other types of study, so that an inspection of the methods used should identify it.

Terms of identification

Either of the terms systematic review or meta-analysis identifies the design. If there is doubt, then the use of a search strategy should provide confirmation. The terms *review* and *narrative review* can refer to a systematic review or to a study with a less complete collection of primary studies. An *overview* usually indicates a collection of systematic reviews, but it can be used for a set of primary studies.

CHAPTER 4

Interpreting the Results

Interpreting the results presented in a paper can be challenging. Large amounts of information from the statistical analyses can be spread across the text, tables, and figures. To simplify the process of interpretation, the initial focus should be on the findings most relevant to the aim or hypothesis being evaluated. This is usually the result highlighted in the Abstract. For example, the key item for a randomised controlled trial (RCT) would be the size of the benefit (or the harm) of the new treatment. It should be accompanied by a test for statistical significance and a confidence interval (these topics are described in the text that follows). Having established the key items, each table and figure can be then approached by asking 'How will these results influence the interpretation of the main findings?' This sequential approach simplifies the process, making it easier to review the large amount of information presented.

The interpretation of the analyses needs an understanding of several important ideas from statistics and epidemiology. These may seem daunting, but they are really quite straightforward. This chapter presents a simple introduction to the following

The Pocket Guide to Critical Appraisal, Second Edition. Iain K. Crombie.
© 2022 John Wiley & Sons Ltd. Published 2022 by John Wiley & Sons Ltd.

terms: measures of effect size, probability, p-values and confidence, bias, and confounding. It also describes some common questionable research practices.

The effect size

In most quantitative research designs the key item is the effect size, the observed difference between two groups. For example, cohort studies compare the frequencies of the outcomes in exposed and non-exposed groups, and clinical trials do so for the treated and the control groups. Case–control studies identify the factor(s) that distinguish cases from controls. What matters is the magnitude of the effect size, how much the two groups differ, with large differences usually being more important than small ones. Several measures are used to quantify the differences between groups, and these are described in the text that follows.

The relative risk

In cohort studies and clinical trials, the effect size is often presented as a relative risk. It compares the frequency of the outcomes in two groups, dividing the rate in the exposed (or treated) group by the rate in the control group. For example, in a cohort study of the risk among women of dying from heart disease, the rate among those who smoked >25 cigarettes per day was 27 deaths per 100 000 per year, and the rate among non-smokers was 5 per 100 000 per year. The relative risk was $27 \div 5 = 5.4$. Therefore, heavy smoking caused a fivefold increase in the risk of heart disease.

The relative risk takes the value 1.0 if there is no difference between the two groups (if the frequency of the outcome was the same in the two groups, dividing the exposed by the non-exposed will yield 1.0). For cohort studies, with an exposure that increases the risk of disease, the relative risk will be greater than 1.0. As a rough guide, a relative risk of 1.2 would be regarded as a small increase in risk, whereas 2.0 is moderate, 5.0 is large, and >10 is very large.

Relative risks can also be less than 1.0. For exposures such as reg-
ular aerobic exercise, which decrease the frequency of heart disease,
the relative risk could be 0.8, corresponding to a 20% reduction in
risk. In clinical trials the interest lies in whether the new treatment
reduces the frequency of an outcome compared to the control. Thus,
a relative risk of 0.8 indicates that the new treatment was slightly better than the control treatment, whereas one of 0.2 would suggest it
was much better and 0.1 would show it was very much better. In contrast, a relative risk of 1.2 would mean that the treatment could be
harmful.

Other ratio measures of risk

Two other measures of risk, the odds ratio and the hazard ratio, are
commonly presented in research papers. These are interpreted in the
same way as the relative risk: the further the estimate is away from
1.0 (either larger or smaller), the greater the effect size. Case–control
studies use the odds ratio because, for technical reasons, they cannot
calculate relative risks. The hazard ratio is a more sophisticated version of measuring risk for cohort studies and clinical trials. It takes
account of the fact that participants may have been followed up for
different lengths of time.

The absolute risk reduction

The absolute risk reduction does not use ratios; it looks at the arith-
metic difference in the frequency of outcomes in the two groups.
In a clinical trial this would be the frequency of the outcome in the
control group minus that in the treated group. This measure can be
more informative than the relative risk because it conveys a better
sense of the potential importance of an exposure or a treatment.
Suppose a new treatment for a serious disease was shown to have
a relative risk of 0.5, reducing the chances of dying by half. If the
disease was had a low mortality, with only 2% of patients dying
from it, then the treatment would reduce the rate from 2 to 1%.
However, if the disease had a mortality rate of 20%, treatment would

reduce the rate to 10%, preventing many more deaths. This example shows that the potential impact of the relative risk depends on the mortality rate of the disease.

Effect size for surveys

Surveys differ from the other research designs in that they only provide estimates of the frequency of certain characteristics in the group studied. For example, it could be the frequency of asthma in a region of England; or it could be the proportion of people who smoke. Thus, the equivalent of the effect size is the size of the proportion. Surveys often compare the frequency among different subgroups, for example the proportion of men and women with asthma. They could also investigate how the frequency of smoking varies by age.

Taking the play of chance into account

All study results are subject to the play of chance. Suppose when one study was completed, a second identical one was carried out. It is very likely that the effect sizes from the two studies would be similar but not identical. (The characteristics of the patients included might differ, and the data collected could contain different measurement errors.) If the study could be replicated hundreds of times, then taking an average of all the effect sizes would remove the impact of the play of chance. In effect, the average would be very close to the true value. Many of the individual effect sizes will be close to the average value, but by chance a few will be far away from it. Thus, when a study produces an interesting finding we need to know whether it could be real or just due to the play of chance. This involves probability and statistical testing, which sound difficult but are fairly straightforward.

Probability

The probability of throwing a six (with a fair six-sided dice) is one in six. The probability of a single ticket winning the national lottery is 1 in 14 million. Probabilities are simply a way of describing how likely it is that an event will happen. They are commonly expressed as decimal fractions, where one in six becomes 0.167. The interpretation of probabilities is straightforward. When an event has a very small probability, e.g. 0.0001, it is very unlikely to happen. When the probability is large, say 0.9, the event is very likely to happen.

Probabilities vary between 0.0 and 1.0, where 0.0 means an event will never happen and 1.0 means it is certain to happen. Thus, the probability that a healthy adult will eventually die is 1.0, because we all die sometime. In contrast the probability of that adult dying tomorrow is less than one in 100 000, i.e. <0.00001. It is not quite zero because some unlikely event, such as being run over by a bus, might just happen. It is very small because rare events are unlikely to happen.

Probabilities are often termed p-values, in which the letter p stands for probability. They can be written as $p = 0.003$ indicating that an event has a 3 in 1000 chance of occurring. Sometimes these probabilities are rounded up to specific thresholds: $p < 0.05$, $p < 0.01$, and $p < 0.001$, corresponding to significant, very significant, and highly significant. For example, $p = 0.003$ would be expressed as $p < 0.01$. This practice is discouraged. It is better to give the exact p-value, as rounding up introduces an approximation that wastes information.

Statistical tests and p-values

Probabilities lie at the heart of statistical tests. The logic behind the calculation of p-values can seem a bit strange, but the approach is chosen because it is the only one that is valid. Consider a clinical trial comparing a new treatment with a conventional one. The first step is to propose that any difference between the treatments is solely due to the play of chance, i.e. that there is really no difference between the treatments. This is commonly called the Null Hypothesis. (It is not what we are hoping for – everyone would want a new treatment to be superior to the conventional one – however, it is the way the logic leads us.) The statistical test then calculates how likely it is that, by chance alone, we would see a difference at least as big as that observed. The test provides us with a probability, a p-value, which tells us how likely it is that the result is due to chance. When this is small (e.g. $p = 0.003$), the result is unlikely to be due to chance. The Null Hypothesis can be rejected, and we can conclude that one treatment is likely to be better than the other. In contrast $p = 0.65$ suggests that chance could be the explanation and we accept the Null Hypothesis.[1]

There is a convenient threshold for the interpretation of p-values: when the p-value is less than 0.05 (i.e. $p < 0.05$) we conclude that chance is not the explanation. The observed effect size is said to be statistically significant. Smaller p-values, say $p < 0.01$ or even $p < 0.001$, indicate it is even less likely that the result was due to chance. These are termed highly and very highly significant, respectively.

The $p < 0.05$ threshold does not correspond to a guarantee. It is sometimes incorrectly used to decide whether a treatment is effective. Such a rule would mean that a treatment with $p = 0.049$ would be judged effective, whereas in another study, one with $p = 0.051$ would be ineffective. The difference between the p-values is tiny, so it would be absurd to claim that one treatment was effective and the other was not. Statistical testing was developed as way of identifying findings that could be interesting, not to prove effectiveness.

When multiple tests of significance are conducted p-values lose their meaning. Suppose many trials were conducted to evaluate a treatment which, in reality, was not effective. Then, by chance alone, a spuriously significant result would occur, on average, once for every 20 significance tests that were conducted. This is because $p = 0.05$ actually says that the observed result could occur by chance one time in 20.

---

[1] *Technical note.* All statistical tests make assumptions about the nature of the data being analysed. Commonly these are that the data points are independent and that they follow a defined distribution, such as the normal distribution. The interpretation of statistical tests and p-values requires that these assumptions are met. Published papers generally do not provide sufficient information to assess the validity of the assumptions, leaving no option but to take it on trust that the statistical tests are being used appropriately.

Confidence intervals

Because of the play of chance, research studies only provide an estimate of the true effect size. With a large study the estimate should be close to the true value, but it is unlikely to be identical to it. The confidence interval indicates a range within which the true value might lie. Conventionally the 95% confidence interval is used: it shows the range within which we are 95% sure that the true size of effect might lie. This can be helpful when deciding whether a treatment is clinically important. For example, a relative risk of 0.4 might have a 95% confidence interval 0.3–0.55. This shows that the true value is most likely in the narrow range 0.3–0.55. However, if the same relative risk had a confidence interval 0.05–0.95, there is considerable uncertainty about what the true value might be. The confidence interval conveys more useful information than p-values.

Factors that distort the effect size

Bias

Bias is the bane of medical research. It occurs when the observed effect size differs from the true value because of systematic flaws in the design or conduct of a study. Unlike random chance, which sometimes pushes the effect size up, and sometimes down, bias consistently pushes it in one direction. The difference between random and systematic errors can be illustrated by considering a digital thermometer that makes errors. If it produces random errors, then some patients will have too high a reading, and for others it will be too low. But when calculating the average for a group of patients, the falsely high and low readings will tend to cancel each other out, so the group average will be close to the true value. If the errors are systematic, either high or low, then the group average will be consistently pushed in one direction.

Random errors become important when comparing two groups. Usually they bias the effect size towards the null (i.e. towards no difference between the groups); the effect appears smaller than it really is. In contrast, systematic errors can either inflate or underestimate the estimated effect size. Most often it is unclear which way the bias will push the effect size. This uncertainty makes it difficult to interpret the study findings.

A large number of biases afflict medical research; a website hosted by the University of Oxford (https://catalogofbias .org) identifies over 60 of them. They can occur in the design, conduct, analysis, and interpretation of studies. Although there are many types of bias, they all act to distort estimates of effect sizes. The biases most common in the different research designs are described in Chapters 6–11.

Confounding

Confounding occurs when part, or all, of the observed association between two variables is due to the action of a third factor. A well-known example of this is the relationship between birth order and Down's syndrome. Studies show that first- and second-born children have a much lower risk of the disease than children further down the birth order. In fact, the relationship is due to the age of the mother, as women having a third or fourth child will usually be older than mothers having a first or second child. Older mothers are at much higher risk, even if they are having their first child. Similarly, the association between alcohol consumption and lung cancer is due to confounding by smoking. Smokers on average drink more, and it is smoking that causes lung cancer.

Confounding is a common feature of surveys, case–control studies, and cohort studies, and even RCTs can be affected. It occurs because many aspects of human health and behaviour are interrelated. For example, with increasing age blood pressure tends to rise, and older people may need glasses to help them read. This does not mean that hypertension causes difficulties in reading. Instead, both are a consequence of ageing. Reducing the impact of confounding is one of the major challenges in medical research.

Confounding is a particular problem for modest relative risks in the range 0.5–2.0. Research has shown that such effect sizes could easily be produced by confounding. In contrast, large effects (relative risks <0.2 or >5) are unlikely to be due solely to confounding. As modest treatment effects are the ones commonly reported in research studies, confounding is often a serious problem.

Questionable research practices

There is substantial evidence that research findings can be distorted by the manipulation of data or the statistical analysis. This may be motivated by the desire to produce more interesting (statistically significant) findings. Three techniques that are commonly used to manufacture spurious p-values are described.

Hypothesising after the analysis

Research studies often collect a large amount of data, although only a small amount is published. The wealth of data means multiple statistical tests can be conducted. Then a chance finding could be presented as if it were a prior hypothesis that was being tested. New study aims could be created, making it appear that the authors showed good judgement in their selection of the research question. This may not be the result of deliberate cheating: subconscious biases could enable the researchers to persuade themselves that they really knew in advance what would be found in the analysis. It can then appear permissible to change the aims.

Detecting changes in the aims is difficult, as it requires access to the protocol for the original study. The protocols of RCTs can be published in journals, or the main study features can be posted on an international register of clinical trials (e.g. International Clinical Trials Registry Platform or clinicaltrials.gov). Checking these sources can identify instances of hypothesis changing. However, for other study designs, such as surveys or cohort studies, few protocols are published and international registries, if available, are seldom used. The only option for critical appraisal is gut feeling: if the hypothesis being tested is somewhat unexpected, to the point of being bizarre, then the study findings should be treated with caution.

Data manipulation

When an initial analysis produces a non-significant finding, the data can be manipulated. One technique is to plot out the data to check whether a few data points are responsible for the lack of statistical significance. The offending points could be removed and the data reanalysed; this process could be continued until the desired (statistically significant) result is obtained. An alternative approach is to alter the unwanted data values to ones that beautify the results. The technical term for this is cheating. It is an egregious practice, but one that is difficult to detect.

Rounding p-values down

A high premium is placed on obtaining statistically significant results. Careful analysis of published p-values shows that there is an excess of p-values just below $p = 0.05$, with a corresponding deficit just above it. It seems that some researchers are nudging non-significant p-values down so, for example, a $p = 0.053$ becomes $p < 0.05$. This behaviour is also difficult to detect. Surveys of statisticians reveal that some have engaged in rounding down p-values, often because of pressure from more senior staff.

Conclusion

The use of p-values and confidence intervals can aid the interpretation of effect sizes. Bias, confounding, and questionable research practices can distort the findings. Large, exciting, and unexpected results are exceedingly rare, whereas flawed studies with misleading findings are much more common. Results should be approached with care, assessing what they mean while looking for possible flaws.

CHAPTER 5

The In-Depth Interrogation

The in-depth interrogation is conducted through questions targeted at key elements of the design, conduct, and interpretation of research studies. Separate sets of questions are provided for each research design (Chapters 6–11). As many of these questions appear in several designs, it is simpler to describe them once here, rather than repeating explanations in subsequent chapters. The questions are organised in two groups: one on bias and the second on value.

Bias

All research designs can suffer from bias; that is, from flaws that systematically distort the findings of a study. Although some research designs (e.g. case–control studies) are more susceptible to it than others (e.g. randomised controlled trials, RCTs), it is best to assume that all studies may be affected by it.

The Pocket Guide to Critical Appraisal, Second Edition. Iain K. Crombie.
© 2022 John Wiley & Sons Ltd. Published 2022 by John Wiley & Sons Ltd.

The questions that assess bias are designed to lead to one of three conclusions: yes, no, or unsure (there is not enough information to decide). With most questions 'yes' means bias is likely and 'no' that bias is unlikely. For clarity of phrasing, the direction of a few questions is reversed, so that the answer 'yes' means bias is unlikely and 'no' that it is unlikely. The interpretation will always be clear from the context and the nature of the bias being assessed.

Research papers should provide sufficient detail for all the answers to be either yes or no. The response unsure signals a potential weakness: the authors may be unaware that this piece of information is important or, possibly, have chosen to omit it. The bias questions are divided into three groups: critical, important, and indicative.

Critical questions for bias

The critical bias questions focus on those elements of a study that, if poorly conducted, place a study at high risk of bias. For each research design, only three or four issues are critical for bias. A flaw detected by any of the critical questions makes the findings suspect.

The critical issues differ across the research designs. For example, adequate adjustment for confounding is critical for case–control and cohort studies but is only an important question for RCTs and surveys. Because of these differences between research designs, the critical questions are not described in this chapter. Instead, they are presented in Chapters 6–11, which deal with the individual research designs.

Important questions for bias

The important questions identify those study elements that could cause substantial bias but are not certain to do so. The findings only become suspect when the study fails on two or three of the important questions. The important questions that apply to most research designs are described in the text that follows; a few further questions are added for the individual research designs in Chapters 6–11.

Is the recruitment strategy clearly described?

Research is conducted on a sample of participants with the aim that these individuals are representative of a larger group. This larger group is often termed the population of interest or the target population. If the sample is well taken, its findings should apply to the population of interest.

To ensure that a biased sample is not obtained, a detailed recruitment strategy should be developed. This should include where the study subjects were recruited from (e.g. the community or through a health care centre) and how they were recruited (e.g. invitation letters or direct personal contact). The type of sampling (e.g. selecting GPs and taking a random sample of their patients) should be described. Selecting participants because they are easy to identify is likely to produce a biased sample. The methods used to contact potential participants should also ensure that no individuals will be overlooked. Information on each of the steps in the recruitment process enables an assessment of the potential for bias.

Are the measurements likely to be valid and reliable?

Poor measuring techniques can lead to substantial errors. The methods of measurements should be discussed, with references given for established procedures. Particular attention should be paid to difficult measurements, such as those involving subjective assessments. Accuracy of measurement can be a problem for lifestyle factors such as diet or physical activity: they are composites of many individual actions and capturing all their facets can be difficult.

Another concern is whether efforts have been made to standardise measurements between observers. In large studies several researchers may collect data and it is important that they have been trained to do so in the same way. A related issue is the sensitivity of the measuring process. A sympathetic interviewer may encourage patients to describe their experiences in full, whereas a more abrasive interviewer might gather much less detail. For example, collecting data on illicit drug use requires an empathic interviewer and a setting in which the participant is comfortable, and confidentiality is guaranteed.

For crucial data items, such as the outcome of an RCT, the method of measurement should be valid and reliable. Validity is the extent to which a method measures what it is supposed to measure. For example, when estimating alcohol consumption, valid answers are unlikely to be obtained to the question 'how much do you drink?' Many study participants will understate their true consumption, although those who are boastful may exaggerate. Research papers should confirm that measures of proven validity are used to obtain data on key data items.

A reliable measure is one that gives a similar result when taken on more than one occasion. For example, the measurement of an adult's height can be affected by many factors. These include the way an individual stands, the angle at which the head is inclined, and whether or not shoes are worn. In general, paper should clarify the steps taken to ensure that a standardised method of measurement was used.

Could missing data be a problem?

Few studies are able to collect complete data on all participants; some questionnaires may not be completed, or problems with the equipment may mean some measurements are not taken. The extent of missing data should be described, and the consequences assessed. In practice, details of the missing information are often only given in footnotes to tables and are seldom discussed in the text. Small amounts of missing data, in the order of a few per cent, are unlikely to distort the main findings, but extensive data loss, say more than 10%, could cause bias. Bias is likely to occur if those who have missing data are different from the other participants (e.g. in terms of age or disease severity).

Are the statistical methods appropriate?

Inappropriate statistical analysis can produce misleading results. All statistical tests make some assumptions about the data being analysed, and it is encouraging when this issue is explicitly addressed. If there is doubt about the appropriateness of the analysis, a statistician should be contacted. One warning sign is the use of exotic statistical tests – was the test selected because of the p-value it yielded? Concern is also raised when the only results presented are those from a sophisticated statistical technique. Simple analyses should be presented first and compared with the more complex ones. If discrepancies are found between the two analyses, they should be explained in the text of the paper. Unexplained discrepancies cast doubt on the propriety of the analysis.

Was the adjustment for confounding adequate?

Most studies investigate the relationships between factors. For example, a cohort study might investigate whether educational attainment at school or college is related to subsequent income. The problem is that any observed relationship could be influenced by other factors, such as lifestyle or mental wellbeing. However, mental wellbeing could affect school performance and this could also affect subsequent income. So, any relationship between educational attainment and income could be influenced by the confounding factor mental wellbeing.

Studies that explore relationships should use statistical models to adjust for (remove) the effects of potential confounders. This will give a more accurate estimate of the strength of the relationship. These methods rely on two assumptions: that all the potential confounders have been identified, and that each has been perfectly measured. The important confounders should be described, and justified, in the Methods section. When obvious confounders have been omitted, the observed relationship could be misleading. The appearance of an unexpected potential confounder in the analysis could suggest it has been included because it helped to give a desired (significant) result.

In practice, it is unlikely that all the relevant confounders are known; the hope is that the important ones are used in the analysis. This leaves the possibility of unmeasured, or residual, confounding, where an unknown factor has modified the effect size. Residual confounding is a particular issue for small effect sizes, such as a relative risk of 1.2. If some important confounders have been poorly measured, or left out of the analysis, the observed effect could be due to the influence of unmeasured or poorly measured confounders. .

Are all the main findings discussed?

The Results section of papers should present all the important findings from the research. Sometimes the Methods section describes data that have been collected but apparently not analysed. This may have an innocent explanation, such as shortage of space, or it could be that an unwelcome finding was not reported. There is an understandable tendency among researchers to draw attention to findings that fit their preconceptions. Results that contradict prior beliefs are sometimes ignored.

Was there data dredging?

Some studies collect data on as many different items as the imagination and resources of the researchers allow. This enables a number of different hypotheses to be tested at the same time. The analysis can trawl through the variables, looking for anything of interest, so that multiple significance testing becomes a major hazard. The calculated p-values can no longer be interpreted at face value, and instances of spurious statistical significance will occur. Researchers may overlook this hazard, persuading themselves that the chance finding was actually what they were looking for. This is known as hindsight bias, in which memory is distorted so that the person misremembers having predicted a particular result.

The problem of multiple testing can be avoided by using appropriate statistical methods to ensure that spuriously significant results do not occur. In practice, these methods are seldom used. It is simpler if studies nominate one primary hypothesis and then conduct a few other tests. In this situation conclusions about statistical significance are only valid for the nominated test; the other tests are considered to be exploratory. If any of the other tests were thought to be of interest, then new studies would have to be conducted to test each one as a primary hypothesis.

Could selective reporting of outcomes have occurred?

Many studies collect data on several outcome measures, one of which has been nominated as the primary hypothesis. If the analysis yields a non-significant result, a different (statistically significant) outcome measure may be reported in a research paper, with the initial one being quietly buried. The technical term for this is cheating. It is a common practice that produces biased findings. There may be circumstances in which outcomes are changed for legitimate reasons, but if so, the authors should state them.

Identifying outcome switching can be difficult, as it involves searching for the study protocol. These documents are often available for clinical trials, and to a lesser extent for systematic reviews, because there are online registries for these research designs. For other designs, such as surveys and cohort studies, locating the documents will be difficult. Selective reporting is an important cause of bias, but one that can be hard to detect.

Has spin been used to mislead?

Spin is reporting studies in a way that is intended to mislead. It comes in many forms. Authors often exaggerate research findings that are weak or inconclusive. They do so because spin can influence the judgement of other researchers. Selective citation of previous studies, in the Introduction and the Discussion, can make the study appear novel. This false impression can be reinforced by using terms such as innovative, ground-breaking, unique, and remarkable. These are weasel words, used to create the impression that the findings are important. Very few studies merit such labels, so these claims should be treated as suspicious.

A common spin technique is to imply that a treatment was beneficial when there was a null finding; the lack of statistical significance can be concealed with phrases such as a trend to significance. Another technique is to highlight a minor finding in the Abstract because it was statistically significant. The Abstract is the part of the paper that is most often read. This may tempt authors to showcase what they consider to be the best result, even if it is not the one that was identified in the stated aims.

The presence of spin could suggest that the authors know that their methods may be flawed or that the findings are unimpressive. Important findings from high-quality studies do not need to be exaggerated. Spinning the interpretation of findings is a common cause of bias and should be sought out so that exaggerated findings can be disregarded.

Could conflict of interest have influenced the findings?

Most journals require authors to declare financial conflicts of interest that might have influenced the design, conduct, or interpretation of the study. These include the receipt of gifts, travel expenses, funding for research, or personal payments. The pharmaceutical industry is noted for its generous giving to researchers. Many people think they are unaffected by this largesse, but it can influence judgement. Gifts induce a sense of obligation and a need to reciprocate, such that judgement is biased in favour of the giver. Conflicts of interest are often not reported, but when they are it is worth inspecting them to see whether they might compromise study quality.

Was there industry involvement in the study?

Studies that are funded by the pharmaceutical industry have a marked tendency to produce results that favour the company's products. It is often suggested that some form of bias may explain these findings. An alternative explanation is that these companies only test drugs for which they have good prior experimental evidence. However, hundreds of millions of pounds (sterling) of profit can be generated by a new effective treatment. Given this magnitude of incentive, it would be prudent to treat industry involvement in a study as a potentially serious conflict of interest.

Indicative questions for bias

Indicative questions are those which suggest that there may be deficiencies in important study elements, but do not identify specific biases. They provide a warning sign, pointing to potential sources of bias.

Are the study aims focused?

The aims of the study should identify the specific research question to be answered. Clearly stated, focused aims suggest that the study has been well planned. In contrast, wide-ranging or vague aims suggest that the study was a fishing expedition that collected large amounts of data that were then subject to extensive analyses. This increases the risk of multiple testing and the possibility of spurious statistical significance.

Was the sample size justified and achieved?

Research should only be carried out when it has a good chance of meeting the study aims. One essential part of this is that the study should be large enough to give an accurate picture of what is going on. Conventionally, the size of effect being sought (for example, the likely difference between two treatments) is specified, together with an estimate of the standard deviation. Then a formal sample size calculation is carried out to determine how big the study should be to detect the specified effect. The details of this calculation should be in the Methods section. If the number of participants recruited is much smaller than the required number, the study is unlikely to be able to fulfil its aims. If a sample size calculation is not presented, the researchers may have guessed how many participants were needed, hoping that the sample would be big enough. This could lead to outcome switching or data dredging if the hopes were not realised.

Was a pilot study conducted?

A feature of all research is that unexpected problems always occur. Potential subjects who seemed to be plentiful are in reality difficult to find. Many of those who can be identified refuse to participate. Some of the items in the study questionnaire produce misleading or unhelpful answers. Collecting specimens (e.g. blood samples) proves difficult in the research setting. Insufficient time has been allocated for the study procedures (e.g. identifying participants, obtaining ethical consent, and collecting and processing the data).

The pilot study provides a method to avoid these problems. It is a small-scale project intended to identify the pitfalls lying in wait for the full study, and to provide a realistic estimate of the time and effort that will be required. Research studies that have not tested their methods in a pilot are more likely to fail to achieve their intended sample size and to have data of poor quality. This could lead to data dredging, selective outcome reporting, and the use of spin.

How are null findings interpreted?

A null finding occurs when a treatment, or exposure, does not significantly affect the outcome measure, i.e. the statistical test yields a non-significant result. This result needs to be interpreted with care. It could mean that there really is no effect; that the treatment does not work. Or the treatment might have a weak effect, but the study was too small to show that it was statistically significant. This uncertainty is measured by the confidence interval, which, for a null finding, will cover the range from possibly beneficial to potentially harmful. Null findings are ambiguous, and the only fair interpretation of a non-significant result is that there is insufficient evidence about effectiveness. The conclusion that the treatment was ineffective is not justified, as it confuses 'evidence of no effect', which is not true, with the actual finding 'no evidence of effect'.

Is the discussion of study limitations helpful?

All studies have some flaws and their impact on the findings should be outlined in the Discussion section. Some authors will be reluctant to expand on serious defects in a study, as this could reduce the chances of publication in a prestigious journal. A common technique is to identify one or two minor issues to distract attention from the major flaws. The discussion of limitations should be treated with some scepticism; it is better for the reader to make their own assessment. The absence of discussion of potentially important weaknesses could mean the study was of high quality, or that serious flaws are being ignored. The safe option is to look again for flaws that might cause bias.

Questions about value

The value of research is measured by its potential to improve the lives of patients or members of the public. This could be by the discovery of a new treatment for a disease, or the identification of a preventable cause of a disease. The value of a research finding depends on several factors, which are explored in the following questions.

Were the participant characteristics and the research setting adequately described?

Research studies aim to generalise their findings to a wider group or population. To facilitate this, the clinical and sociodemographic characteristics of the study participant (such as age, sex, or disease severity) should be presented. Many clinical trials exclude patients who are older, or have comorbidities, restricting the extent to which the findings can be generalised. If the nature of the participants is not described, then it will be unclear to whom the findings apply, and the study may have little value.

The research setting is also important. For example, a clinical trial could be conducted in a hospital that is a world leader for care of a particular disease, or it could have been in a general hospital. The setting could influence the observed effectiveness of the treatment, depending on the availability of specialist clinical expertise and of facilities for diagnosis, such as CT scanners. These factors could restrict the generalisability of the findings.

Was the outcome measure important to patients?

Outcome measures should deliver benefits that patients find important. Length of life is clearly important, but so are other issues such as symptom relief, quality of life (such as coping with everyday tasks), emotional and physical wellbeing, and the ability to work. Ideally, researchers will have developed the outcome measure in consultation with patients. In practice, many studies use proxy (surrogate) outcomes such as shrinkage of a tumour (instead of survival or quality of life) or bone mineral density (instead of number of factures or ability to walk). These measures may be related to more important outcomes (such as mortality or functional ability), but often surrogate outcomes may only be weakly associated with patient-important outcomes. Their use reduces the value of the findings.

Was the effect size large enough to be important?

The clinical importance of a result depends on the effect size. Statistical significance is a not a good measure of the value of a finding. A p-value of $p < 0.001$ could occur with a small effect size if the sample size was large. Judging the magnitude of benefit is a subjective process, although rules of thumb have been proposed: a relative risk of 1.2 would be regarded as small increase in risk, whereas 2.0 is moderate, 5.0 is large, and >10 is very large. However, the question of what is a worthwhile effect size will also depend on the context of the study. A treatment that increases the survival of severely ill babies by a few per cent would be worthwhile. In contrast, a small change in the frequency of symptoms such as headache would be less important.

The relative risk can be interpreted from two perspectives: that of the individual, or that of the whole population. For example, most people would choose to avoid an exposure that might double their risk of having a serious disease. But at the societal level the question is different; it focuses on the burden of disease in the population that is due to the exposure. This depends on the frequency of the disease in the unexposed group as well as the relative risk. Suppose that each year 1000 people suffer a serious disease, such a heart attack. A new exposure that doubles that risk would increase the number of cases to 2000 and could put a serious strain on the health care system. In contrast, if only 5 people normally get the disease, then doubling the risk would only increase the caseload to 10. From the population perspective, the background frequency of disease should be taken into account when assessing the value of relative risks.

Was precision assessed?

Most medical journals prefer confidence intervals to p-values because they show the range within which the true value could lie (see Chapter 4). This range is referred to as the precision of the effect size: it allows an assessment of how large or small the true effect might be. A wide range indicates that there is considerable uncertainty about what the true value might be, and the size of effect is considered to have low precision. In this case, the confidence interval should be inspected to determine just how small the true effect size might be.

A helpful approach is to compare the lower estimate of the confidence interval with the smallest treatment benefit that would be thought clinically worthwhile. For example, a reduction of 10% in the mortality rate of patients with high blood pressure might be considered worthwhile, whereas <10% might not. If, for this example, the confidence interval was 15–35%, then even the lower estimate (15%) indicates the benefit was greater than the minimum clinically worthwhile value of 10%. However, if the confidence interval was 4–44%, then the true treatment effect could be as low as 4%, much less than the minimum clinically worthwhile benefit (10%). The precision gives much more information about the value of a treatment than the effect size.

How plausible are the main findings?

A finding can be given more weight when other findings support it. Suppose a cohort study investigated three levels of exposure: low, moderate, and high. Then the finding that the moderate exposure carried a risk that was intermediate between those of the low and high levels would increase the plausibility. This is called a dose–response relationship. Results are also more believable if there is a credible mechanism by which the intervention/exposure achieves its effect. Caution is also needed with this assessment because the biological processes that lead to disease are complex. If knowledge is incomplete, an incorrect disease mechanism may be used to support a misleading finding.

How do the results compare with previous reports?

The results of any study need to be interpreted in the light of previous research. Research findings only achieve general acceptance when supported by several other studies, preferably from more than one research group. Confidence in a finding is diminished if studies by other research groups fail to confirm the result.

Published papers should explain how their findings fit with existing research. This is not always done well. Some authors may be tempted to ignore studies with contradictory results. Others may fail to mention studies with similar findings so that they can claim that their own results are novel. It can be difficult for those not familiar with a particular field to compare a study with previous reports. If the new research appears important, a literature review may be needed to assess its value.

Conclusion

This chapter has described most of the appraisal questions that explore bias and value. Chapters 6–11 present the complete checklists for the appraisal of the common quantitative research designs. These lists will include the critical questions for bias. Sometimes, a question identified as important for bias in this chapter may be promoted to a critical one because the issue is crucial for that design. For example, adjustment for confounding becomes a critical question for cohort and case–control studies. In addition, in some chapters a few new questions are added to the list of the important questions of bias. For example, several new questions are added to the chapter on RCTs. Chapter 6, the first on individual research designs, outlines how to appraise surveys.

CHAPTER 6

Appraising Surveys

This chapter explores the issues that are relevant to surveys that were not covered by the in-depth interrogation questions described in Chapter 5. A list of all the questions of bias (critical, important, and indicative) and those for value is presented at the end of the chapter. The complete set of questions provides a comprehensive guide to the appraisal of surveys.

The critical bias questions for bias

Surveys provide information about groups of people. They take samples of subjects, such as patients, health professionals, or members of the general population. For example, a study may identify a sample of patients with asthma to establish how many smoke. The data are used to estimate the frequency of smoking among patients with asthma in a larger target population. The idea is that a well-taken sample provides a good estimate of the frequency in that larger population. Surveys appear easy to conduct, so they are

The Pocket Guide to Critical Appraisal, Second Edition. Iain K. Crombie.
© 2022 John Wiley & Sons Ltd. Published 2022 by John Wiley & Sons Ltd.

widely used and often misused. Three questions are critical for the risk of bias in surveys.

Will the sampling strategy produce a representative sample?

Surveys take samples to estimate how common things are. An unrepresentative survey will produce a biased estimate. To ensure the sample is representative of the larger population, the stages from identifying the target population to recruiting the participants should be described. For example, if the survey investigated patients with asthma, the target populations could be patients seen in general practice, or those attending a hospital clinic. It could also focus on a subset of asthma patients, such as children aged 16–18 years, adults over 65, or only those with moderate to severe asthma symptoms. The sampling strategy should reflect the larger target population.

The key issue in sampling is that everyone who is considered eligible for the study should have an equal chance of being selected for the sample. Commonly a list of all subjects in the target population is obtained. This is called the sampling frame. Individuals are then selected using a set of random numbers to produce the sample, a process called simple random sampling. Other sampling techniques can be used, such as stratified sampling or cluster sampling. These divide the target population into groups, from which subsamples are taken using simple random sampling.

Many types of sampling frames (lists) are available, but none of them is perfect. The electoral register should cover the entire population, although homeless people and those who do not wish to vote may be missing. Lists of patients registered with GPs also cover most people, although those who move to a different town or city may not be contactable if they have not registered with a new practice. Gaps in the sampling frame can cause bias because some individuals in the target population have no opportunity to be included in the sample.

Some studies recruit subjects because they were easy to contact. This is called convenience sampling. It will be biased because the factors that make people easy to reach will also make them unrepresentative. An extreme form of this is the use of volunteers. Those who come forward to take part in research are likely to differ in sociodemographic factors, and in their experiences of illness, from those who are reluctant to participate. Although bias is certain, the nature of it is unknown. This makes it difficult to generalise the findings.

Is the response rate acceptable?

In surveys some subjects cannot be contacted, and others may refuse to take part. Failure to contact could occur for many reasons: individuals have moved home, have been admitted to long-term care, or have emigrated or died. Those who refuse may dislike filling in questionnaires (or taking part in interviews), have some personal antipathy to the topic being investigated, or have difficulty reading. In addition, older people, those who are socially disadvantaged, and those with mental health problems may be hard to reach. The amount of the bias caused by non-response depends on the number and the characteristics of the non-responders. The size of the sample provides no protection against this bias: if it occurs, response bias will have as great an effect on a study with one million participants as it will on one of 500.

There is no simple rule for an acceptable response rate: some say at least 60%; others 70% or even 80%. Studies that do not give the response rate, or claim a near-perfect response, should be regarded with suspicion. Possibly more important than the response rate is the extent to which the participants and the non-responders differ. Even if the response rate were high, substantial bias could occur if the non-responders were markedly different.

Papers that report survey results should describe the strategies that were used to reduce non-response. They should also discuss how many were missed and what effect this might have on the results. Ideally, a comparison would be made of the characteristics of those who did and did not take part in the study. Failure to address these issues suggests that non-response bias may be a problem.

Are the measurements likely to be valid and reliable?

The issue of the validity and reliability of the data that were collected is a major concern for surveys, so it is treated as a critical item. Surveys commonly collect large amounts of information on hundreds of participants, creating the potential for poor-quality data. Validity and reliability were described in Chapter 5, so that discussion is not repeated here. The important point is that the methods of data collection should be carefully reviewed to determine whether inadequate measurement techniques could introduce bias. If questionnaires were used, their sources, and whether they have been validated, should be stated. If physical or biochemical measurements were taken, details should be given of the instruments used and the procedures followed. Standardisation of measurement techniques should provide valid and reliable data.

The complete list for appraising surveys*

* The questions in italics are the standard ones that were described in Chapter 5.

The critical questions for bias

Will the sampling strategy produce a representative sample?
Is the response rate acceptable?
Are the measurements likely to be valid and reliable?

The important questions for bias

Is the recruitment strategy clearly described?
Could missing data be a problem?
Are the statistical methods appropriate?
Was the adjustment for confounding adequate?
Are all the main findings discussed?

Was there data dredging?
Could selective reporting of outcomes have occurred?
Has spin been used to mislead?
Could conflict of interest have influenced the findings?
Was there industry involvement in the study?

The indicative questions for bias

Are the study aims focused?
Was the sample size justified and achieved?
Was a pilot study conducted?
How are null findings interpreted?
Is the discussion of study limitations helpful?

Questions of value

Were the participant characteristics and the research setting adequately described?
Was the outcome measure important to patients or the general public?
Was the effect size large enough to be important?
Was precision assessed?
How plausible are the main findings?
How do the results compare with previous reports?

CHAPTER 7

Appraising Cohort Studies

This chapter explores the issues that are relevant to cohort studies that were not covered by the detailed interrogation questions described in Chapter 5. A list of all the questions of bias (critical, important, and indicative) and those for value is presented at the end of the chapter. The complete set of questions provides a comprehensive guide to the appraisal of cohort studies.

The critical questions for bias

Cohort studies follow study participants through time to determine what happens to them. The aim may be to follow the natural time course of disease, or to determine whether risk behaviours (e.g. excessive alcohol consumption) or environmental exposure (e.g. to industrial chemicals or air pollution) can increase the risk of disease. Four questions are critical for the risk of bias in cohort studies.

The Pocket Guide to Critical Appraisal, Second Edition. Iain K. Crombie.
© 2022 John Wiley & Sons Ltd. Published 2022 by John Wiley & Sons Ltd.

Was an appropriate control group used?

Cohort studies that monitor prognosis of disease do not need a control group, but those that evaluate exposures that may cause harm require controls. Suppose the cancer risk of industrial pollution was being assessed. The frequency of cancer in the exposed group would need to be compared with that in a control group to determine whether there was an increased risk.

The key issue is whether the control group is sufficiently similar to the exposed group to enable a fair comparison to be made. A good control group resembles the study group on factors such as age, gender, and lifestyle, differing only on exposure. One way to increase the chances of suitability is to recruit participants from the same source population. For example, the classic cohort study on smoking and lung cancer obtained subjects from the register of British doctors, dividing them into smokers and non-smokers. If the two groups are selected from different source populations, bias is likely.

Similarity between the two groups can also be increased by matching each exposed individual to an unexposed one. The matching uses the baseline factors that might be associated with the outcome measures. Commonly the two groups are matched for age and gender, but other factors, such as such as area of residence, could also be used. This approach reduces the risk of bias from confounding factors.

Another concern is the response rate – the proportion of those invited to take part in the study who are successfully recruited. A difference in frequency of participation between the two groups could bias the estimated effect size. Even if recruited from the same source population, unequal response rates could lead to differences in the characteristics of the two groups. All cohort studies should compare the sociodemographic characteristics of the two groups at recruitment to determine whether they are sufficiently similar for a fair comparison to be made.

Could there be errors in assessing exposure status?

A key issue for cohort studies is that all those allocated to the exposed group really were exposed and that no one in the control group was exposed. Incorrectly allocating exposed individuals to the control group, or unexposed ones to the exposed group, will cause bias. This is commonly described as misclassification bias. Suppose a study investigated the impact of air pollution (the exposure) in a local area on the frequency of asthma attacks (the outcome). If some individuals were identified as being in the local area (exposed) when they were elsewhere, the estimate of the effect size could be biased.

The impact of the bias depends on how much misclassification occurred in those in those who suffered an asthma attack compared with those who did not. If the frequency of misclassification is the same in those who had an attack as in those who did not, then the effect size will be biased to the null (towards no association between exposure and outcome).

The consequences of this bias are different when the frequency of misclassification is related to the outcome measure. For example, if it was higher frequency in those who had an asthma attack than those who did not then the direction of this bias is uncertain; the effect size could be pushed upwards or downwards. (The same uncertainty about the direction of the bias will occur if the frequency of misclassification is lower in the asthma sufferers than those free from asthma.) Misclassification could occur if knowledge of the outcome influenced the measurement of the exposure. The question to ask is whether knowledge of the outcome could influence the measurement of exposure. Published papers should provide details of how exposure was measured, and the steps taken to prevent misclassification of the exposure measurement.

Were the outcomes measured in the same way for the exposed and the control groups?

The outcomes in cohort study can be events such as death, or occurrence of a serious disease. These are commonly measured using routinely collected data that can be accessed by researchers with legitimate interests. Physiological or biochemical measures of disease status, like peak flow for respiratory disease or plasma creatinine for renal disease, also provide objective measures. The research staff measuring these outcomes should be blind to (unaware of) the exposure group of the participants.

Many outcomes, such as mental wellbeing or chronic pain, require the completion of validated questionnaires. These raise the concern of whether the exposed group and the control group completed the questionnaires in the same way. If assessed by interview, care is needed to ensure that those collecting the information are unaware of whether the participant is in the exposed or control group, otherwise bias might occur. Knowledge of the exposure status could affect the nature of the questioning, possibly encouraging more probing for the exposed group, biasing the assessment of the outcome.

Could loss to follow-up be a problem?

In follow-up studies patients have many opportunities to disappear. Moving house, death, emigration, or admission to a long-stay hospital can all result in study participants being lost to follow-up. Whatever the reasons, those lost to follow-up are likely to differ from those who remain in view. The greater the extent of this loss, the greater the potential for bias. A common rule of thumb is that the loss of <5% is unlikely to cause bias, whereas >20% is problematic. A particular concern is with differential loss to follow-up: if more subjects are lost from one exposure group than the other, then bias is likely.

The characteristics of those lost to follow-up are also important. For example, if many of those with high levels of exposure were lost, then the estimated effect of exposure would be underestimated. Another concern is whether loss to follow-up is due to the loss of certain types of individuals. This can be assessed by comparing the baseline characteristics of those who were lost with those successfully followed up. The analysis should be conducted separately for the exposed and the control groups to determine whether loss to follow-up could introduce bias. If this information is not provided, the risk of bias is uncertain.

Follow-up rates can be increased, by contacting participants a few times asking them to get in touch if they move house. Sending reminders just before the date of follow-up and making repeat attempts to contact those who have been missed can also help.

Failure to use any strategy to improve follow-up is a warning sign that bias could be introduced by incomplete follow-up.

Was the adjustment for confounding adequate?

Cohort studies are particularly susceptible to confounding, making the adequacy of adjustment a critical issue. The problem is that exposures are often correlated with other factors that can also affect the occurrence of the disease. For example, suppose a study was carried out to investigate the health consequences of heavy alcohol consumption. Those who overindulge could differ from moderate drinkers and abstainers in factors such as smoking, diet, physical activity, and occupation. Adjustment for all these factors would need to be made in the statistical analysis as they could also affect health outcomes. The key question is whether all the important potential confounders have been identified, and whether they have been accurately measured. Failure to adjust adequately for these factors could bias the effect size, making it appear larger than it really is. This phenomenon is called residual confounding, in which part of the observed effect size is due to insufficient adjustment for confounders. The concern is that a complete adjustment for the confounders could have shown that the exposure had no effect on the outcome. Residual confounding is always possible in cohort studies.

The important questions for bias

Was the length of follow-up adequate?

The length of follow-up should be reviewed to clarify whether the study had a reasonable chance of detecting important events. The minimum length of follow-up depends on the exposure being studied. For example, in a study of asthma and air pollution, a few days of follow-up would be sufficient to detect the outcomes. However, in a smoking and lung cancer study, many years of follow-up would be needed to detect the association between exposure and outcome.

If the follow-up period is too short the estimated effect size will underestimate the true impact of exposure. This is a concern for studies in which very few events were observed, as this could happen if the length of follow-up was insufficient.

Did the analysis allow for the passage of time?

When cohort studies follow people up for several years, individuals in one group may have an average length of follow-up that is larger than that of the other group. This could occur if more people are lost from one group (say the control) than from the other (the intervention). Even when loss to follow-up is similar in the two groups, a difference in average follow-up times will occur if more individuals drop out earlier (i.e. die or are lost to follow-up) in one group than the other. Having similar average follow-up times is important because the longer the follow-up the more disease that will occur. This could happen if, for example, more of those in the exposed group died before the follow-up was completed. Imbalance will create differences between the frequencies of disease in the two groups, biasing the relative risk. Statistical methods can adjust for this and these should be described in the Methods section of the paper. It may be difficult for the non-statistician to be sure if the methods are truly appropriate, but it will be possible to check that some attempt has been made to cope with this complexity.

The indicative questions for risk of bias

Was the study prospective or retrospective in design?

Prospective cohort studies contact potential participants and follow them up for a specified time into the future. This enables detailed information to be collected on the baseline characteristics of the participants. In contrast, retrospective studies identify subjects from some time in the past using registers such as the employee records of industrial companies or patient records of health care organisations. These individuals are then followed up to the present day.

This can mean that the information on the key item, the exposure, is not collected with the same accuracy as in a prospective study. In addition, the amount of baseline data that can be obtained from the records is often limited so that adjustment for confounding may be inadequate. Retrospective cohort studies may be at a higher risk of bias, so the quality of the exposure data and the adequacy of adjustment for confounding should be carefully reviewed.

The complete list for the appraisal of cohort studies*

*Items in italics are the appraisal questions that were described in Chapter 5.

Critical questions for bias

Was an appropriate control group used?
Could there be errors in assessing exposure status?
Were the outcomes measured in the same way for the exposed and the control groups?
Could loss to follow-up be a problem?
Was the adjustment for confounding adequate?

Important questions for bias

Is the recruitment strategy clearly described?
Are the measurements likely to be valid and reliable?
Could missing data be a problem?
Are the statistical methods appropriate?
Was the length of follow-up adequate?
Did the analysis allow for the passage of time?
Are all the main findings discussed?
Was there data dredging?
Could selective reporting of outcomes have occurred?
Has spin been used to mislead?

Could conflict of interest have influenced the findings?
Was there industry involvement in the study?

Indicative questions of risk of bias

Are the study aims focused?
Was the sample size justified and achieved?
Was the study prospective or retrospective in design?
Was a pilot study conducted?
How are null findings interpreted?
Is the discussion of study limitations helpful?

Questions of value

Were the participant characteristics and the research setting adequately described?
Was the outcome measure important to patients or the general public?
Was the effect size large enough to be important?
Was precision assessed?
How plausible are the main findings?
How do the results compare with previous reports?

CHAPTER 8

Appraising Case–Control Studies

This chapter explores the issues that are relevant to case–control studies that were not covered by the detailed interrogation questions described in Chapter 5. A list of all the questions of bias (critical, important, and indicative) and those for value is presented at the end of the chapter. The complete set of questions provides a comprehensive guide to the appraisal of case–control studies.

The critical questions for bias

Case–control studies often investigate why certain people develop a specific illness. They can also investigate why some patients behave as they do; for example, why some do not attend for cervical screening. These studies identify a group of individuals (the cases) who have a disease or other characteristic of interest, such as not attending for cervical screening. These individuals are then compared with a group of people, the controls, who do not have the

The Pocket Guide to Critical Appraisal, Second Edition. Iain K. Crombie.
© 2022 John Wiley & Sons Ltd. Published 2022 by John Wiley & Sons Ltd.

disease (or characteristic of interest). The study looks backwards in time to determine which factors in the past could explain why one group of individuals became cases and the other did not. The method appears straightforward, but case–control studies are more susceptible to bias than many other research designs. Four questions are critical for the bias of case–control studies.

Was the identification and recruitment of cases clearly described and systematic?

To ensure that only true cases are identified, the definition of a case should be clearly stated. For example, in studies investigating potential causes of lung cancer, this would be the diagnostic criteria that identify this disease. The recruitment method should describe the source from which participants were selected and the time period of recruitment. The aim should be to include all the eligible cases (or a random sample of the cases) from that source. A grab sample of cases opportunistically recruited from several sources (a few from here, a few from there) could produce a biased estimate of the effect size.

Is the control group appropriate?

Selecting appropriate controls is one of the major challenges of case–control studies. The intention is that the controls should resemble the cases in all ways, except that they do not have the disease (or characteristic of interest). In general, the two groups should be similar in terms of age, sex, social class, and area of residence. Controls are usually selected from the same source, and over the same time period, as the cases. Ideally, the cases and the controls should be representative samples from the same population.

A key design feature is that the eligibility criteria (for inclusion and exclusion) that were used for cases should also be used for the controls. For example, in a study of the causes of chronic obstructive pulmonary disease (COPD), the cases could be non-smoking men aged over 50 years. Then the controls should be similar, except for not having COPD. Equally, if patients with allergic diseases (such as eczema and asthma) were excluded from the cases, then this restriction should also apply to the controls.

Were data on potential risk factors collected in the same way for cases and controls?

Case–control studies commonly collect many data items, such as the demographic characteristics of the participants (age, gender, and socioeconomic status), together with lifestyle and any other factors that could be related to the likelihood of becoming a case. This information could be obtained by interviews, case-note searches, or postal questionnaires. The details of the data collection techniques need to be scrutinised to confirm they were identical for cases and controls. The same questions should be used, with similar probing for clarification in interviews or equal scrutiny of case-notes.

A particular concern is whether awareness of which individuals were cases and which controls could bias the collection of risk factor data. The depth of probing in interviews or searching through case-notes could be greater if the researcher collecting the data knew that a participant was a case. Blinding to case/control status should be used where possible.

Was the adjustment for confounding adequate?

Case–control studies are particularly susceptible to confounding. Adjustment for confounding can reduce the amount of bias. Papers on case–control studies should carefully review potential confounders and describe the statistical methods used to adjust for them. The results for both the unadjusted and the adjusted analyses should be presented, with an assessment of the impact of the adjustment on the effect size. When the investigation and discussion of confounding is minimal, or obvious confounders are not included, bias is highly likely.

The important questions for bias

Were incident cases used?

Cases fall into two groups: those that have newly diagnosed disease (incident cases), and those with a longstanding illness (prevalent cases). Those with longstanding disease may not be representative of all cases because some patients who had the disease may have been cured or have died. Selective loss of some cases could introduce bias. For example, those who died could have had adverse health behaviours, such as heavy smoking or other serious illness. This would mean that the surviving cases were on average healthier than incident ones. The direction of the bias with prevalent cases is unpredictable, either overestimating or underestimating the effect size. It is better to use incident cases.

Could ascertainment bias be a problem?

Ascertainment (or detection) bias can occur when extraneous factors make it more likely that a case is identified and included in a study. For example, suppose a study wanted to investigate a link between smoking and the skin cancer malignant melanoma. Smokers generally visit their GPs more often than non-smokers (for conditions such as for bronchitis and emphysema) and may have an early-stage melanoma diagnosed while attending for some other reason. These incidental diagnoses will increase the proportion of smokers among the cases, creating a spurious association between smoking and melanoma.

Prior knowledge of the exposure could also influence the recruitment of cases, biasing the estimated effect size. This could happen when medical records are being reviewed to identify potential cases. Suppose there was uncertainty over whether a specific patient, a potential case, had the disease of interest. Knowing that the individual had been exposed to the risk factor could be used to confirm that the individual was a case. This can happen when the same source (e.g. case-notes) is used to identify cases and to obtain data on exposure: while searching for information on the diagnostic criteria the researcher may come across details of the exposure.

Were the response rates different for cases and controls?

Bias can occur during the recruitment of cases and controls if there are differences in the response rates (the proportions of those contacted who agreed to participate). For example, in a study of obesity some potential cases might be reluctant to take part because of sensitivities about their weight. The control group would not have these concerns and might have a higher response rate. However, in a study on the causes of breast cancer, those with the disease may be more willing to participate because they want to know why they became ill. Bias is likely if one group has a much lower response rate than the other. To investigate this, the characteristics of responders and non-responders could be compared, with the results for the cases and controls presented separately.

Could misclassification bias have occurred?

Misclassification bias can occur when some individuals are incorrectly identified as cases, or if some who were thought to be controls were actually cases. This bias can occur when the definition of cases is not sufficiently clear: the supposed case may not have the disease of interest but suffer instead from a condition that resembles it. For example, endometrial hyperplasia could be misclassified as frank carcinoma. Then any factors associated with hyperplasia (e.g. exogenous oestrogens) would be falsely associated with the cancer. It is difficult to detect whether this bias has occurred; the best that can be done is to review the definitions of cases and controls to determine whether they are sufficiently detailed and do not contain ambiguous phrases.

Could recall bias be a problem?

Many case–control studies obtain data by interviews with the study participants. Bias can occur if there are differences in the recall of past events between cases and controls. For example, if the cases are patients with serious illness, they may answer questions differently from healthier controls. Those with severe disease often reflect on their history to try to understand why they became ill. They are likely to remember events more clearly, and in greater detail, than the controls. This is usually described as recall bias, in which members of one group provide more detailed information than the other.

Is there a plausible interval between exposure and diagnosis of disease?

Exposures to noxious substances can take different lengths of time to cause disease. For example, the latency period for nutritional deficiency diseases such a scurvy and beriberi ranges from a few weeks to a few months, whereas calcium deficiency only leads to osteoporosis after several years. If there is information about the mechanism of disease causation, or the natural history of a disease, it may be possible to specify a likely interval between exposure and diagnosis. In the absence of such clues, the chosen interval between exposure and diagnosis may be little more than a guess. Studies in which the interval is too short may underestimate the effect size, or even fail to identify any association between exposure and disease.

The complete list for the appraisal of case–control studies*

* The questions in italics are the standard ones that were described in Chapter 5.

The critical questions for bias

Was the identification and recruitment of cases clearly described and systematic?
Is the control group appropriate?
Were data on potential risk factors collected the same way for cases and controls?
Was the adjustment for confounding adequate?

The important questions for bias

Were incident cases used?
Could ascertainment bias be a problem?
Were the response rates different for cases and controls?

Are the measurements likely to be valid and reliable?
Could misclassification bias have occurred?
Could recall bias be a problem?
Could missing data be a problem?
Is there a plausible interval between exposure and disease?
Are the statistical methods appropriate?
Are all the main findings discussed?
Was there data dredging?
Could selective reporting of outcomes have occurred?
Has spin been used to mislead?
Could conflict of interest have influenced the findings?
Was there industry involvement in the study?

The indicative questions for bias

Are the study aims focused?
Was the sample size justified and achieved?
Was a pilot study conducted?
How are null findings interpreted?
Is the discussion of study limitations helpful?

The questions of value

Were the participant characteristics and the research setting adequately described?
Was the outcome measure important to patients or the general public?
Was the effect size large enough to be important?
Was precision assessed?
How plausible are the main findings?
How do the results compare with previous reports?

CHAPTER 9

Appraising Randomised Controlled Trials

This chapter explores the issues that are relevant to randomised controlled trials (RCTs) that were not covered by the detailed interrogation questions described in Chapter 5. A list of all the questions of bias (critical, important, and indicative) and those for value is presented at the end of the chapter. The complete set of questions provides a comprehensive guide to the appraisal of RCTs.

The critical questions for bias

The RCT is a type of controlled experiment that tests whether one treatment produces a better health outcome than another. It provides the most rigorous and reliable method for evaluating effectiveness of health care interventions. The most common type of RCT has two groups: one receiving the new intervention (treatment group), and

The Pocket Guide to Critical Appraisal, Second Edition. Iain K. Crombie.
© 2022 John Wiley & Sons Ltd. Published 2022 by John Wiley & Sons Ltd.

the other a standard intervention (control group). Four questions are critical for bias in RCTs.

Were patients randomly allocated to treatments?

The aim of random allocation is to produce two groups of patients who are similar at baseline (at the start of the study). This enables a fair comparison of the outcomes of the two treatments. Computer-generated random numbers are used to create the sequence in which patients will be allocated to treatments. This ensures that each patient has the same chance of being allocated to the new treatment as they do of becoming a control. The randomness will, on average, produce comparable groups. The process of generating the random sequence should always be described. It is best if the random allocation is conducted in conjunction with an independent clinical trials unit.

Not all clinical trials use random allocation and it may not be possible to make a fair comparison of treatments. The term quasi-randomised is a warning signal – it usually means that patients have been allocated to treatments using a method that is convenient for the researchers, such as day of admission to hospital or by even or odd dates of birth. These methods are predictable and could enable a motivated person to meddle with the sequence in which patients were allocated to treatments. Tampering with the randomisation sequence will cause bias.

Was the allocation to treatments concealed?

Efforts should be made to conceal the group to which each patient is allocated from the health care staff who recruit the patients. The aim is to prevent clinicians or researchers from altering the sequence in which patients are given treatments. Suppose a clinician, about to enter a new patient into a trial, thought that a patient should receive the intervention (new) treatment. If the patient had been allocated to the control treatment, the doctor might decide to exclude them from the study. Selectively excluding some patients could bias the results. Trials with inadequate or poorly described methods of concealment often produce inflated estimates of the benefits of the intervention (compared to studies with high-quality concealment). Poor allocation concealment is one of the main causes of bias in randomised trials.

Could lack of blinding bias the assessment of the outcome?

Bias can be introduced into the outcome assessment if any of the following groups know which treatment the patients received: the clinicians managing the patients, the patients reporting the outcomes, the researchers measuring the outcome, or the statistician analysing the data. A caring physician who thought one treatment was less effective might compensate by giving more care and attention to patients receiving it. Patients who believe they are getting an expensive new drug may report being better than they really are. The researcher might, through some misplaced enthusiasm for the trial, subconsciously nudge the measurements to favour the new treatment. A statistician could be tempted to search the data for some difference that would support one of the therapies. To prevent bias, the patient, clinician, researcher, and statistician should be blind to treatments given.

Could loss to follow-up be a source of bias?

In clinical trials, contact with some patients may be lost during the follow-up period. The concern is whether the patients who disappear are special in any way. For example, if the new treatment was effective, some patients may fail to attend a scheduled appointment because they have completely recovered and do not see a need to attend. Alternatively, if the new treatment was less effective, some patients could be so ill that they are unable to travel to their appointment. Whatever the reason, selective loss of patients will bias the estimate of treatment benefit.

The amount of bias increases when large numbers of those who were randomised are not included in the analysis of the outcome.

A rule of thumb for losses to follow-up is that <5% loss is unlikely to cause bias and that >20% loss is serious, with those between 5 and 20% being problematic. Concern is heightened if more patients are lost from one treatment group than the other, as this suggests there could be selective loss of patients.

When loss to follow-up is likely to be a problem, the technique of multiple imputation can be used to estimate the missing outcome data. Properly conducted multiple imputation can overcome the bias that loss to follow-up can cause. (This is a sophisticated statistical process that is beyond the scope of this book.) An alternative but inappropriate technique, last case carried forward, is commonly used to compensate for missing outcome data. This method has been widely criticised because it is more likely to cause bias than to prevent it. Current guidance is that the use of this technique indicates that a trial is at high risk of bias.

Have the outcomes been selectively reported?

Many trials collect data on several outcome measures. Such studies should nominate one outcome as the primary one that is used to measure the effectiveness of the intervention. The other outcome measures are classed as secondary and are used to help interpret the findings from the primary outcome rather than to test effectiveness. For example they may shed light on the mechanism of action of the treatment. Studies that do not designate primary and secondary outcomes could engage in multiple testing, presenting only the results for the outcome that gave statistically significant results.

Recent research has shown that the primary outcome reported in published papers often differs from that identified in study protocols. Sometimes this may be done for good reasons. For example, the outcome might be changed if it proved difficult to collect accurate data on the original one. But outcome switching and selective presentation can be done to mislead. A common technique is to replace the non-significant primary outcome with a statistically significant secondary one. The intended primary outcome is demoted to secondary status or even completely ignored. Sometimes an outcome measure that was not mentioned in the protocol displaces the primary outcome. These substitutions often favour outcomes that have large effect sizes and are statistically significant. This results in an overestimate of the benefit of treatment. Uncovering this type of bias is time consuming: it involves searching for the study protocol or the trial registration details to compare with the published report. In many instances this information will not be available. Selective outcome reporting is an important but difficult to detect source of bias.

The important questions for bias

Was the trial registered or was a protocol published?

Researchers are strongly encouraged to register their trial in one of the several international registries that have been established (e.g. International Clinical Trials Registry Platform and clinicaltrials.gov). This should be done before the first patient is recruited to the study. The aim of registration is to promote trial quality: the existence of an easily accessible online record of the methods is intended to discourage changes to the methods during the conduct of the study. Compared with registered studies, unregistered trials have poorer methodology and report larger effect sizes. Studies that are registered will state this clearly, so those that do not mention registration are likely to be at high risk of bias.

In addition to registration, the study protocols are often published in medical journals or made available online. These provide additional information about the methods and the data analysis, making it easier to check changes in study details. Registration and publication of protocols provide some protection against unplanned alterations to the methodology. However, they do not provide a guarantee: many trials that have been registered, or have made available the full protocol, still make changes to the primary outcome or the statistical analysis.

Were the treatment groups comparable at baseline?

Random allocation of treatments is used to guard against bias in assigning patients to treatments. However, this technique does not guarantee that the two treatment groups will be identical at the start of the study. By chance, a few more of the severely ill patients could be allocated to one group than the other. Non-comparable groups could also occur because of problems with the randomisation process, particularly inadequate concealment of the allocation schedule.

When the groups are unequal at baseline, the estimate of the effect size could be biased. Statistical adjustment for confounding factors can reduce the impact of baseline differences between groups. If there are potentially important differences between the groups, and no adjustment has been made, the effect size may be biased. All trials should report the baseline characteristics of the intervention and control groups and should comment on any differences that were observed.

Did the treatment and control groups receive similar care?

Apart from the intervention being studied, the treatment and control groups should receive the same level of care. Deviation from equal care is termed performance bias. It could occur if the study protocol states that one group should have more follow-up visits than the other. More visits would provide the patients with more opportunities to report symptoms and would give the clinician more opportunities to order investigations or to prescribe additional drugs. Similarly, if one group received more tests, or counselling and general support, then the effect size could be biased. Any differences in ancillary care may cause bias.

Performance bias could also occur if the health care team managing a patient was aware of the treatment being given. If the treatment was thought to be inferior or to carry a higher risk of adverse effects, additional care might be given to the patient. This could lead to bias. Ensuring that the healthcare staff were blind to treatment group could prevent this.

Was the length of follow-up adequate?

The length of follow-up will depend on the disease being treated and the effect of the treatment. For example, patients with infectious diseases commonly recover after a few days, sometimes weeks, of antibiotic treatment. In contrast, patients with depression or rheumatoid arthritis may need to take drugs for months or years. For these patients the follow-up period should be long enough to be clinically meaningful. A short interval could fail to detect the benefit from the treatment. Alternatively, it could detect a short-term benefit that was not sustained, leading to an overestimate of the true value. The length of the follow-up interval should be justified.

Were the outcomes clearly defined, and measured in the same way for intervention and control groups?

Bias could occur if there were differences between the groups in the way the outcomes were measured. Those making the measurements should receive the same training in the use of the data collection instrument (questionnaire or device/equipment) and the data should be collected in similar settings (clinic or home). Although published papers often do not give this level of detail, it is important to be sure that any differences in outcomes between intervention and control were not a consequence of differences in measuring techniques.

Were the results analysed by intention to treat?

In the course of an RCT, patients may have their treatments changed and may even swap from one treatment to the other. Whatever has happened, the recommended approach is to analyse the study by the groups to which the patients were first allocated (intention to treat). This approach reflects what will happen when the treatment is used in routine care, where treatment changes often occur.

An alternative approach, per-protocol analysis, excludes those patients who did not receive the intended treatments. This includes those who missed a few treatments or had their treatment changed. The argument is that estimates of effectiveness could be misleading if some patients did not receive the full course of treatment. There is some merit in this. The problem is that per-protocol analysis ignores the concern that patients whose treatment is changed, or who are withdrawn from the study, may be systematically different to those who do not change. Excluding these patients from the analysis could introduce differences between the two groups, and the comparison of treatments would no longer be fair. The consensus is that per-protocol analysis is likely to cause more bias than intention to treat. The per-protocol method of analysis is strongly discouraged.

A more extreme version of per-protocol analysis is modified intention to treat (mITT). It involves excluding patients from the analysis for various, often dubious reasons. The term has no agreed definition. Studies that use it should be treated as being at very high risk of bias.

Could small sample size be a problem?

Trials with small numbers of patients often produce exaggerated estimates of treatment benefits. In many instances the findings of these studies are subsequently refuted when additional RCTs are conducted. These exaggerated findings can be due to the play of chance, such that out of the multitude of small trials, a few will produce aberrantly large effect sizes.

Small trials are particularly vulnerable to baseline imbalance, making them more susceptible to confounding. If only 50 or so patients have been recruited, imbalance at baseline is highly likely, and adjustment for confounding may be unable to remedy this problem. (For technical reasons, confounding can only adjust for one or two confounders if the sample size is small. This limits the amount of adjustment for confounding, leaving the studies at risk of bias.) RCTs with small sample sizes and unexpectedly large effect sizes are potentially unreliable.

The questions of value

All the value questions for RCTs were covered in Chapter 5, except for one on harms.

Have data on harms been presented and discussed?

Many treatments have unwanted side effects: amoxicillin can cause nausea and diarrhoea, amitriptyline causes dry mouth and sedation, and surgical operations certainly have their hazards. When assessing value, the beneficial effect of a therapy has to be balanced against its side effects, taking account of their frequency and severity.

Identifying harms is difficult. The side effects of treatments are often not known, and novel or unexpected side effects may not be recognised. As RCTs commonly have fewer than 100 patients and have relatively short follow-ups, rare and long-term harms may not be detected. The adverse events that are detected during the conduct of trials are often under-reported in published reports. When they are reported, the studies sometimes give the total number of patients with side effects, with no information on the severity of these effects. In some instances, the adverse effects are simply described as being tolerable or acceptable. The lack of data on the frequency and severity of the adverse events means the benefit to harm ratio cannot be evaluated, leaving the value of the treatment uncertain.

The complete list for the appraisal of clinical trials*

* The questions in italics are the standard ones that were described in Chapter 5.

The critical questions for bias

Were patients randomly allocated to treatments?
Was the allocation to treatments concealed?
Could lack of blinding bias the assessment of the outcome?
Could loss to follow-up be a source of bias?
Have the outcomes been selectively reported?

The important questions for bias

Was the trial registered or was a protocol published?
Is the recruitment strategy clearly described?

Are the measurements likely to be valid and reliable?
Were the treatment and control groups comparable at baseline?
Did the treatment and control groups receive similar care?
Was the length of follow-up adequate?
Were the outcomes clearly defined, and measured in the same way for intervention and control groups?
Could missing data be a problem?
Were the results analysed by intention to treat?
Are the statistical methods appropriate?
Was the adjustment for confounding adequate?
Could small sample size be a problem?
Are all the main findings discussed?
Was there data dredging?
Has spin been used to mislead?
Could conflict of interest have influenced the findings?
Was there industry involvement in the study?

The indicative questions for bias

Are the study aims focused?
Was the sample size justified and achieved?
Was a pilot study conducted?
How are null findings interpreted?
Is the discussion of study limitations helpful?

Questions of value

Were the participant characteristics and the research setting adequately described?
Was the outcome measure important to patients?
Was the effect size large enough to be important?
Was precision assessed?
Have data on harms been presented and discussed?
How plausible are the findings?
How do the results compare with previous reports?

CHAPTER 10

Cohort Studies That Evaluate the Effectiveness of Interventions

Cohort studies are increasingly used to evaluate the effectiveness of treatments. The widespread availability of electronic health record systems has accelerated the use of this type of study. These record systems were originally designed to assist clinical staff in delivering care and to enable administrators to manage health care resources efficiently. They provide doctors with rapid access to patients' previous medical histories including episodes of illness, diagnoses, laboratory test results, treatments, and subsequent outcomes. They also enable administrators to monitor resource use and reduce health care costs. It is now widely recognised that these databases offer many advantages for medical research. However, this type of cohort study also suffers from many flaws and biases that limit the value of its findings.

The Pocket Guide to Critical Appraisal, Second Edition. Iain K. Crombie.
© 2022 John Wiley & Sons Ltd. Published 2022 by John Wiley & Sons Ltd.

This chapter begins with a brief review of the advantages offered by this research design and the challenges for critically appraising it. For convenience the abbreviation 'cohort treatment study' will be used for this research design. The chapter also describes some of the factors that make it difficult to conduct critical appraisals, and then reviews the questions that assess risk of bias and value.

Overview of advantages of cohort treatment studies and challenges for critical appraisal

Advantages

The advantages of cohort treatment studies lie in the ease with which they can be conducted. The use of electronic health records allows large numbers of patients to be identified, and the subsequent outcomes can be measured easily and at low cost. The large sample sizes provide estimates of treatment effect that have high precision and can also detect rare adverse effects. By undertaking extended follow-ups using historical data, this method can also identify long-term benefits and harms of treatments. In addition, these studies can be used in circumstances where when very few randomised controlled trials (RCTs) have evaluated a particular treatment, or when it may not be feasible or ethical to conduct an RCT.

Another benefit of cohort treatment studies is their ability to measure the effectiveness of treatments as they are used in routine clinical care. A limitation of RCTs is that they are often conducted in carefully controlled conditions on selected, closely monitored groups of patients. The characteristics of the patients seen in clinical practice may differ from those in RCTs: they may be older, have more comorbidities, or adhere less well to the treatment schedule than those who were included in the RCT. The phrase real-world evidence is now widely used to emphasise the ability of cohort studies to evaluate treatments as they are used in clinical practice. Many national and international medicines regulatory authorities are developing guidance for the use of real-world evidence in making decisions about health care delivery. Countries around the world are making substantial investment in the technology and infrastructure to foster this research into the effectiveness of treatments.

Challenges for critical appraisal

Assessing the risk of bias in cohort treatment studies is often hampered by the poor quality of reporting of study methods in published papers. There are guidelines for the reporting of cohort studies. (Strengthening the Reporting of Observational Studies in Epidemiology [STROBE], and more recently REporting of studies Conducted using Observational Routinely-collected health Data [RECORD]. The latter addresses topics such as data cleaning and access to study protocols and to the raw data that are not covered in STROBE.) These reporting guidelines are not regularly required by medical journals and are often not followed. In contrast, adherence to the guidelines for RCTs (Consolidated Standards of Reporting Trials [CONSORT]) is required by most journals.

The poor reporting of methods is compounded by very low rates of study registration and the limited availability of study protocols. (This contrasts with RCTs, where registration of study methods is frequently required and protocols are widely available.) It is difficult to compare the intended methods with those described in the published paper, so unplanned changes to the outcome measures or the statistical analysis cannot be detected. In addition, the limited descriptions of key methodological details often lead to the answer 'not sure/not enough information' to the appraisal questions. This uncertainty about the risk of bias is a major weakness of cohort treatment studies.

The critical questions for bias

Cohort treatment studies compare the outcomes among patients given one treatment (the intervention group) with those of patients given a different treatment (the control group). They are at risk of the same sources of bias as conventional cohort studies, but also suffer from some additional biases. The first question examines the many problems of data quality that plague cohort treatment studies. Subsequent questions explore the biases that occur because patients are not randomised to treatment and the strategies that can be used to lessen their impact.

Were efforts made to improve data quality and were these methods transparent and reproducible?

The quality of the data in electronic health records is a major concern. It is salutary to compare the accuracy of the data in RCTs with that in electronic health records. When RCTs are conducted, considerable effort and a large amount of the funding are devoted to ensuring that the data are complete and accurate. Trained research staff apply specific diagnostic criteria to recruit patients and use specially designed questionnaires to collect baseline and outcome data. In contrast routine health care data are processed by administrative staff who are unaware of the research study and of the diagnostic criteria and the outcome assessments that it will use. Clinical data are collected and coded to be useful for administrative purposes and the management of patients, not for research.

Incomplete or inaccurate data are common in large electronic databases. Errors frequently occur in patient characteristics, their diagnoses, the treatments prescribed, and the outcomes recorded. Male patients recorded as being admitted to gynaecology or obstetrics wards is one example of the errors that can occur. The frequency of errors can be reduced by data cleaning: identifying missing data, out-of-range values (e.g. a patient aged 150 years), or logical inconsistencies (patient prescribed a drug but no record of it being administered). One strategy is to delete the cases with missing or incorrect data items, although this only conceals rather than rectifying the problem. A better alternative is to use other pieces of information about the patients to derive new values for missing or illogical data points. Machine learning algorithms are increasingly being used to facilitate this. Despite many efforts to improve quality, concerns remain that errors in the data could introduce bias.

The important issue for critical appraisal is that efforts were made to improve data quality. The methods should be clearly described, with references to studies that assessed the validity of the techniques used. Particular attention should be given to key data items: the diagnosis and its date, the treatment given with the start date, and outcome measures. If appropriate techniques have been employed, the data may be of moderate to high quality; without them it is likely to be poor.

Could the process of selecting treatments for patients bias the estimates of effect size?

In cohort treatment studies, patients meeting specific diagnostic criteria are identified but are not randomised to treatment groups. Instead, their doctors select treatments based on the patients' clinical characteristics, such as the duration and severity of the disease and the presence of comorbidities. There will often be good clinical reasons why some patients received one treatment and others were given a different one. For example:

- patients who become seriously ill might be given a more aggressive treatment;
- those who were elderly, frail, or in poor health may be given a milder treatment;
- those who did not respond well to a previous treatment might be swapped to a new or expensive one;
- patients with a family history of a disease could be given a different treatment to other patients.

The way treatments are allocated to patients makes it likely that the intervention and control groups will be systematically different at baseline (i.e. at the start of the study). The outcomes may be affected by these differences, making it difficult to determine what impact the treatments had. This phenomenon is sometimes called 'confounding by indication'. It occurs when an observed outcome is not due to the treatment given but to the reasons (the indications) that the treatment was given to a group. For example, patients with severe disease might have been given drug A, while those with milder symptoms were given drug B. Any difference between the outcomes of the two treatment groups could be due to the initial severity of disease and not to the treatments.

Was the control treatment chosen to minimise confounding by indication?

The bias caused by non-random allocation of treatments could be reduced by careful choice of the control group. At issue are the indications for intervention and control treatments – the clinical factors that led to the treatments being chosen. If these are similar, it is likely that the two groups of patients will be comparable. When the two treatments have different indications, the patients they are given to are likely to be different. The greater the divergence between the clinical indications, the more the baseline characteristics of the two groups will differ. The issues of clinical indications, and the suitability of the control treatment, should be carefully addressed. If they are ignored, there is likely to be potential for confounding by indication.

Were efforts made to reduce or adjust for confounding?

Cohort treatment studies are very susceptible to confounding because patients are not randomised to treatment group. The strategies that were used to minimise this risk should be clearly described. The effects of confounding can be reduced by incorporating either of two design features, restriction or matching. Restriction identifies the main confounder and only recruits patients who are similar on that factor. For example, if hypertension were important, the study could focus on patients with moderate hypertension (or severe hypertension).

Matching involves assessing the confounding factors for each patient in the treatment group, then finding a patient in the control group who has similar characteristics. For example, if age, obesity, and disease severity were confounders, each patient in the intervention group would be matched to a control who was similar on these three factors. These strategies should be justified in the paper.

An alternative approach is to adjust for confounding in the analysis. The statistical techniques and the confounding factors to be included should be described and justified. The possibility that residual or unmeasured confounding may have influenced the observed effect size should also be discussed. Failure to address these issues suggests that the estimated treatment effect may be biased.

The important questions for bias

Was the study hypothesis testing or exploratory?

Hypothesis testing studies nominate in advance the two treatments to be compared and the primary outcome that will be used to assess effectiveness. The p-values and confidence intervals can be legitimately assessed. In contrast, exploratory studies commonly compare several different pairs of treatments and can use a variety of outcome measures. Their aim is to identify potentially interesting associations between treatments and outcomes. Confidence intervals and p-values can be calculated but, because of multiple significant testing, they have little worth. An interesting finding from an exploratory study needs to be assessed in a hypothesis testing study to determine whether the observed effect is important or spurious.

Problems arise when an exploratory study is presented as if it were a hypothesis testing one. When carefully written, it can be difficult to determine that the study was not a hypothesis testing one. A plausible justification for the study could be created retrospectively and the methods, including the sample size calculation, could be described as if they had been pre-specified. Many treatment–outcome pairs may be investigated until a statistically significant effect size is uncovered. The possibility that a particular result was carefully selected from a large number of uninteresting ones is a serious concern in cohort treatment studies. Exploratory analyses are only legitimate if the authors report exactly what was done and acknowledge the major weakness that stems from multiple significance testing.

Were the same inclusion and exclusion criteria used for the intervention and control groups?

In cohort treatment studies, all the patients are recruited from the same database of electronic health records. The inclusion (diagnostic) criteria and the reasons for exclusion (e.g. presence of certain comorbidities) should be the same for intervention and control patients. Applying the exclusion criteria with more vigour to one group than the other could lead to differences between the two groups. Bias could also occur if, for one of the two groups, some patients were excluded from the study because of their baseline characteristics (e.g. age or disease severity). This could occur during the data cleaning phase of the study. It is difficult to detect these sources of bias.

Could immortal time bias be a problem?

A well-publicised cohort study found that actors who were awarded Oscars lived longer than those who did not achieve this honour. Although intriguing, the finding is misleading. To win an Oscar, the actor must live long enough to attend the ceremony at which the award is given. In contrast, actors who do not win Oscars can die at any time. For the winners, the period before the award is called immortal time, because, by definition, these actors cannot die before receiving their Oscar.

A good example of immortal time bias is the effectiveness of inhaled corticosteroids for the treatment of chronic obstructive pulmonary disease (COPD) following discharge from hospital. A cohort study could follow up patients from their date of discharge, comparing the survival of those who received the drug against those who did not. As there is often a delay of a few weeks between discharge and the prescribing of the inhaled corticosteroids, patients must live long enough after discharge to receive a prescription. For them this interval is immortal time, with the amount of bias depending on the average length of the time to receipt of the drug. In general, this bias can be identified by asking whether entry into one of the groups will be delayed – whether there is a time-related criterion for being in that group. This could be receiving a prescription, having an operation, or winning an Oscar.

The questions of value

One of the value questions that was covered in Chapter 5 poses a particular challenge for cohort treatment studies and is reviewed in the text that follows. All the other questions of value were dealt with in Chapter 5.

Was the outcome measure important to patients?

A weakness of electronic health records is that standardised, validated outcome measures that are important to patients are seldom used. Instead, studies have to rely on the data items that have been collected for administrative and clinical purposes. Some outcomes, such as death, will always be recorded but it is unlikely that other patient-relevant outcomes will be available (such as symptom relief, quality of life, emotional and physical wellbeing, and the ability to work). A major weakness of cohort intervention studies is that, although they provide real-world evidence, the findings may not be important to patients.

Conclusion

Cohort studies that test the effectiveness of treatment have the potential to provide real-world evidence, particularly in circumstances where few RCTs have been conducted. Five factors substantially weaken that evidence: the poor quality of the data, the bias that results from the way treatments are selected for patients, the limited extent of adjustment for confounding, the opportunities for selective reporting of outcomes, and the limited relevance of outcome measures to patients. In addition, because of limitations in the available descriptions of study design and conduct, there will often be considerable uncertainty about many other potential sources of bias. Research intended to develop improved methodologies is currently underway and may, in the future, overcome some of the weaknesses of cohort treatment studies. At present, all that can be fairly concluded is that for many studies the risk of bias is likely to be high. However, when the intervention and control group treatments have similar indications and the data quality is high, the risk of bias may be low.

The complete list for the appraisal of cohort studies that evaluate interventions

This list is a combination of the appraisal questions presented in this chapter with some from Chapters 5 ('The In-Depth Interrogation'), 7 ('Appraising Cohort Studies'), and 9 ('Appraising Randomised Controlled Trials'). The questions from these three chapters are in italics. Those from Chapter 5 are distinguished by the symbol *, those from Chapter 8 by a †, and those from Chapter 9 by the symbol Φ. The questions that are new or have been substantially modified from the version in previous chapters are in plain text.

Critical questions for bias

Were efforts made to improve data quality and were these methods transparent and reproducible?
Could the process of selecting treatments for patients bias the estimates of effect size?
Was the control treatment chosen to minimise confounding by indication?
Were efforts made to reduce or adjust for confounding?
Could loss to follow-up be a problem?†
*Could selective reporting of outcomes have occurred?**

Important questions for bias

Was the study registered or was a protocol published?Φ
Was the study hypothesis testing or exploratory?

Were the same inclusion and exclusion criteria used for the intervention and control groups?
*Are the measurements likely to be valid and reliable?**
*Could missing data be a problem?**
*Are the statistical methods appropriate?**
Was the length of follow-up adequate?†
Did the analysis allow for the passage of time?†
Could immortal time bias be a problem?
*Are all the main findings discussed?**
*Was there data dredging?**
*Could selective reporting of outcomes have occurred?**
*Has spin been used to mislead?**
*Could conflict of interest have influenced the findings?**
*Was there industry involvement in the study?**

Indicative questions of risk of bias

*Are the study aims focused?**
*Was the sample size justified and achieved?**
*How are null findings interpreted?**
*Is the discussion of study limitations helpful?**

Questions of value

*Were the participant characteristics and the research setting adequately described?**
Was the outcome measure important to patients?
*Was the effect size large enough to be important?**
*Was precision assessed?**
*How plausible are the main findings?**
*How do the results compare with previous reports?**

CHAPTER 11

Appraising Systematic Reviews

This chapter explores the issues that are relevant to systematic reviews that were not covered by the detailed interrogation questions described in Chapter 5. A list of all the questions of bias (critical, important, and indicative) and those for value is presented at the end of the chapter. The complete set of questions provides a comprehensive guide to the appraisal of systematic reviews.

The critical questions for risk of bias

Systematic reviews aim to provide a comprehensive, unbiased summary of all the studies on a focused clinical question. They achieve this by systematically searching for relevant research studies, evaluating the quality of individual studies, and summarising the findings. The term primary studies is used for the set of studies that meet the criteria for inclusion in the systematic review. Commonly, the effect sizes from the primary studies are combined using meta-analysis.

The Pocket Guide to Critical Appraisal, Second Edition. Iain K. Crombie.
© 2022 John Wiley & Sons Ltd. Published 2022 by John Wiley & Sons Ltd.

This is a statistical technique that pools the effect sizes from the relevant studies to give an overall estimate of treatment effect. It produces an estimate that has a much higher precision than any of the individual studies.

Systematic reviews and meta-analyses of medical treatments play a prominent role in the development of clinical practice guidelines, so they need to be of high quality. They suffer from several flaws that can place them at risk of bias. Five critical questions can help reveal the main weaknesses.

Was the search strategy adequate?

The strength of systematic reviews is that they summarise the findings from all the studies relevant to the research question. To achieve comprehensive coverage a detailed search strategy covering several sources of studies should be developed. The four key elements of a search strategy are the: Patient group, Intervention group, Comparison group, and Outcome measure (PICO). If these components are not well described, the review is at risk of bias.

Most clinical research studies are indexed in electronic databases such as MEDLINE, EMBASE, and CINAHL. Computerised searches of these databases form the backbone of systematic reviews. The review should specify which databases were searched and it is recommended that at least three databases are used. Combinations of search terms for each of the PICO components are organised in a logical sequence to form the search strategy. The search terms comprise keywords (in normal English) and standardised subject terms that are provided by each database. For example, MEDLINE indexes papers using MeSH terms (Medical Subject Headings), whereas EMBASE uses Emtree. Both provide an extensive vocabulary of terms that are organised in a hierarchical tree structure. These standardised terms provide an efficient method for extensive and consistent searching of the databases, and frequently identify studies that normal English words might miss. Review studies should provide a full description of the search strategy. Those that mention only a few keywords or do not use MeSH or Emtree terms may overlook many relevant studies.

In addition to electronic databases, other sources, commonly termed the grey literature, are often searched. This can involve hand searching of the reference lists of key papers, reviewing studies published in selected journals, and examining conference abstracts. In addition, experts can be asked to nominate relevant studies. The absence of these extended searches could mean that relevant studies may have been missed.

In summary, high-quality search strategies use well-developed searches based on the PICO model, involve at least three electronic databases, and complement these with searches of the grey literature. The absence of a detailed, comprehensive search indicates that the review may be more haphazard than systematic.

Was publication bias assessed?

Small studies and those with unimpressive findings are much less likely to be published than large studies or those with statistically significant findings. This is publication bias. The concern about unpublished studies is that their findings might be consistently different from those that were published. When only published studies are included in the review, the summary estimates often exaggerate the true treatment effect.

Systematic reviews should explore whether there might be publication bias. A graphical technique, the funnel plot, and statistical methods, such as trim-and-fill, can help identify publication bias. When these tests suggest there is bias, the reviewers should conduct additional literature searches, particularly of the grey literature. If publication bias is not assessed, it is possible that the summary estimate will be biased. In this event, the direction and magnitude of bias can only be guessed at, making conclusions unreliable.

Was the risk of bias of the primary studies taken into account?

A major strength of a systematic review is that by pooling data from all relevant (primary) studies it provides an estimate of treatment effect that has much higher precision than the individual studies. However, some of the studies may be at high risk of bias, which could distort the pooled estimate. Systematic reviews should assess the quality of the studies selected for inclusion.

Many systematic reviews assess the risk of bias of the individual studies, then ignore the findings and include all the studies in the analysis irrespective of their quality. This defeats the purpose of assessing bias. An alternative approach, excluding poor-quality studies from the analysis, could be wasteful of information. A better approach is to conduct sensitivity analyses. This involves an initial pooling of the results with all the primary studies. Then those at the highest risk of bias are excluded and the analysis is repeated. A comparison of the two analyses would indicate how sensitive the findings are to the inclusion of studies at high risk of bias. Both analyses would be presented with appropriate cautionary remarks if the two pooled estimates differed markedly. Conclusions should be based on the findings from the analysis that excluded the studies at high risk of bias. Failure to assess the quality of primary studies, or assessing it but ignoring it, places the findings of systematic reviews in doubt.

Was heterogeneity of effect fully investigated?

The studies included in the systematic review are likely to have slightly different effect sizes. This could be due to differences in the design and conduct of the individual studies. The common sources of variation are: the characteristics of participants (clinical, sociodemographic, or lifestyle factors); design features such as the dose and duration of treatment, adequacy of blinding, and concealment of treatment allocation; and the definition of the outcome and the way it was measured. Together these factors cause heterogeneity (differences in effect sizes of the individual studies).

The extent of heterogeneity can be assessed by statistical indices such as the I-squared statistic, I^2. This measures the proportion of the variation in treatment effects that is due to differences in methodology between studies (rather than to chance). A rough guide to the interpretation of I^2 is that 25% might indicate mild heterogeneity, 50% is moderate, and 75% is substantial. Formal statistical tests can also be used to determine whether the amount of variation is greater than would be expected by chance. If these yield small p-values (e.g. $p < 0.01$) then heterogeneity is likely.

Systematic reviews should investigate heterogeneity by exploring whether the individual effect sizes are scattered across a wide range. Concern is increased if some studies find large beneficial effects and others harmful effects. The extent to which the confidence intervals overlap should also be examined: if there is little overlap, then substantial heterogeneity is likely.

When heterogeneity is suspected, statistical techniques (meta-regression models) can be used to explore which design features might explain it. These will show the amount of heterogeneity that remains (residual heterogeneity) after adjusting for the design features. The challenges that heterogeneity creates should be explicitly acknowledged in the Discussion section.

Was an appropriate method used to combine estimated effect sizes?

Many systematic reviews pool the results of individual studies, using the methods of meta-analysis. However, when there is clear evidence of substantial heterogeneity, a meta-analysis may produce biased or wholly misleading findings. Instead, a narrative review could be conducted, in which the findings from the primary studies are discussed. Formal methods, such as combining p-values or vote counting based on direction of effect, can assist in drawing general conclusions. Vote counting based on statistical significance is strongly discouraged.

When pooling of studies is appropriate, two methods can be used: fixed effects models and random effects models. Fixed effects models are simpler, but they ignore heterogeneity. If there is diversity in the characteristics of the primary trials and there is evidence of heterogeneity (e.g. the I^2 is large), the pooled estimates from these analyses may be misleading or even meaningless.

Random effects models incorporate unexplained heterogeneity into the model and the pooled effect size will usually have wider confidence intervals. This model assumes that the individual studies are estimating different effects that are distributed around a central value. The question of when to use fixed effects or random effects models has been widely debated but remains unresolved. It is recommended that both methods be used, and their results compared.

The important questions for risk of bias

Were the papers carefully screened for inclusion?

Thorough searching for papers usually identifies large numbers of potentially relevant studies that need to be screened using well-defined, unambiguous selection criteria. The criteria are usually based on the PICO components (Patient group, Intervention, Comparison group and Outcome measure), but may include other elements such as the study designs to be included (e.g. randomised controlled trial [RCT] or cohort) or the time period (in years) in which the studies were published. The criteria should be inspected carefully: imprecise criteria could lead to a heterogeneous group of studies; over-restrictive criteria could exclude relevant studies.

Screening the long list of potentially relevant studies is usually conducted in two stages. Initially, titles and abstracts are inspected to identify studies that appear appropriate. Then the full texts of these papers are obtained and carefully reviewed, leading to one set of relevant papers for inclusion and a further set of those to be excluded. This second stage should be conducted independently by two reviewers. Sufficient detail should be given to make the screening process explicit and reproducible; inadequate reporting suggests that the methods may be poor.

Were the data extracted by more than one reviewer?

The extraction of key items from the primary studies (particularly the effect size, its standard deviation, and the sample size) is prone to error. To minimise this, data extraction should be conducted independently by at least two reviewers, with discrepancies resolved by discussion. If this process of data extraction is not mentioned, errors may distort the overall effect size or its confidence interval.

Was missing information sought?

Sometimes, information on some key methodological details is not contained in the published papers. This could make it difficult to assess the quality of a study or, in some instances, could lead to a study being excluded from the systematic review. Reviewers will often write to the study authors requesting these details. If this is not done, some studies may be excluded from the analysis, potentially biasing the results.

How were multiple outcome measures dealt with?

Clinical trials often measure several outcomes. Across all the trials of a particular treatment identified in a systematic review, dozens of different outcome measures may be available for analysis. This could result in cherry picking, where specific outcomes are selected because they give a desired result (i.e. a statistically significant one). To prevent this, the outcome measures should be specified in advance. The chosen outcomes should be justified, with the main criteria being relevance to patients, clinicians, and health care decision makers. It is recommended that a few outcomes are nominated as critical, usually one to measure benefit and another for harm. Several other outcome measures thought to be important can also be included. Failure to address the problem of the multiplicity of outcomes, or the absence of a justification for the choices made, suggests that selective outcome reporting may have occurred.

Could conflict of interest have influenced the findings?

Conflict of interest could affect two groups of individuals: the researchers who undertook the review and those who conducted the primary studies included in the review. The authors of reviews often have direct links with companies that make pharmaceutical and medical devices. There are many stages in the conduct of a review, such as the selection of studies for inclusion and the interpretation of the findings, which require judgement. When conflicts of interest occur, systematic reviews often have conclusions that favour commercial companies.

Conflict of interest among the authors of the studies selected for inclusion presents an additional problem. Trials where authors have conflicts of interest are more likely than other trials to produce positive findings. Inclusion of these studies could bias systematic review findings. The Cochrane Collaboration, which produces authoritative guidance on the conduct of systematic reviews, states that the sources of funding and author conflict of interest should be reported for all included trials. Further, a judgement should be made about the possible consequences of any conflicts. It is not enough to report conflicts of interest – reviews should assess whether they might bias the findings.

The questions of value

There are two questions of value questions for systematic reviews in addition to those covered in Chapter 5.

Has diversity in patients and research settings across the primary studies been assessed?

Marked differences across the included studies in the characteristics of the patients and of the research settings will affect value. This raises the questions of to whom and in what circumstances do the findings apply. Reviews should assess whether the extent of diversity among patients and settings permits firm conclusions to be drawn.

Have data on harms been presented and discussed?

Systematic reviews of RCTs often provide inadequate information on harms. Published trials frequently underreport adverse effects, and systematic reviews sometimes do not include harms data described in trial reports. The guidance for systematic reviews is that data on harms should be presented for each included study. The frequency and severity of harms should be reviewed, together with an assessment of the balance between benefits and harms. Ideally, when the information on harms in the published trials is inadequate, the authors of these studies should be contacted to obtain further details. Failure to discuss harms or the benefit to harm ratio markedly reduces the value of the findings of the systematic review.

The complete list for the appraisal of systematic reviews*

* The questions in italics are the standard ones that were described in Chapter 5.

The critical questions for risk of bias

Was the search strategy adequate?
Was publication bias assessed?
Was the risk of bias of the primary studies taken into account?
Was heterogeneity of effect fully investigated?
Was an appropriate method used to combine estimated effect sizes?

The important questions for risk of bias

Were the papers carefully screened for inclusion?
Were the data extracted by two reviewers?
Was missing information sought?
How were multiple outcome measures dealt with?
Are all the main findings discussed?
Was there data dredging?
How were multiple outcomes dealt with?
Has spin been used to mislead?

Could conflict of interest have influenced the findings?
Was there industry involvement in the study?

The indicative questions for risk of bias

Are the study aims focused?
Was a pilot study conducted?
How are null findings interpreted?
Is the discussion of study limitations helpful?

Questions of value

Were the participant characteristics and the research setting adequately described?
Has diversity in patients and research settings across the primary studies been assessed?
Was the outcome measure important to patients or the general public?
Was the effect size large enough to be important?
Was precision assessed?
Have data on harms been presented and discussed?
How plausible are the findings?
How do the results compare with previous reports?

CHAPTER 12

Summarising Risk of Bias

Previous chapters have presented lists of questions to assess the risk of bias in published studies. This chapter describes a method of combining the resulting information to provide an overall evaluation of the risk of bias. The process is conducted in three steps. The first identifies the potential for bias inherent in each research design. Then the sources of bias in the way the study was designed, conducted, and interpreted are reviewed. Finally, these two assessments are combined to produce an overall risk of bias score.

Identify the risk of bias of the research designs

The research designs can be arranged in a sequence by their susceptibility to bias (Table 12.1). Randomised controlled trials (RCTs) are placed near the top of the list because randomisation enables an unbiased assessment of treatment effectiveness. Systematic reviews, which combine the findings of several RCTs, are placed at the top

The Pocket Guide to Critical Appraisal, Second Edition. Iain K. Crombie.
© 2022 John Wiley & Sons Ltd. Published 2022 by John Wiley & Sons Ltd.

TABLE 12.1   Initial ranking of the research designs.

Design	Risk of bias
Systematic review of RCTs	Low
Randomised clinical trial	Low
Systematic review of cohort and case–control studies	Moderate/high
Cohort study	High
Case–control study	High
Surveys	High
Case series, commentaries, expert opinion, editorials	Very high

because they can greatly reduce the impact of the play of chance. Concerns about confounding and errors in the measurement of exposures and outcomes leads to cohort studies being assigned the level below RCTs. Case–control studies are in the next lowest level because they are conducted retrospectively (backwards in time from the outcome to the risk factors). Surveys, which do not provide estimates of effect size, are ranked lower still. For completeness, case series, commentaries, expert opinions, and editorials are also shown in Table 12.1. These types of study are placed at the bottom because they are at very high risk of bias.

This sequence assumes that the individual studies are of high quality. In addition, for systematic reviews, the risk of bias of the primary studies is assumed to be low. Individual studies only merit their place if they have been carefully designed and executed.

Review the biases in study design, conduct, and interpretation

Care is needed to assess the potential impact of the biases identified by the appraisal questions. It is easy to find flaws in the study design and methods. Research is never perfect; it just needs to be good enough to make bias unlikely. Even in high-quality studies some measurements will be missed, or some participants will drop out. The challenge is to distinguish major flaws from minor hiccups in the research process. Four questions can help identify the serious defects.

- How could this flaw bias the result, and what is the likely mechanism of action?
- How much bias could this type of defect cause?
- Would the bias inflate or underestimate the effect size?
- Could the size and direction of the bias change the interpretation of the result?

Personal judgement is then used to rate each source of bias on a three-point scale: low, moderate, and high. It is helpful to make a list of the potential sources of bias. Having the complete set of assessments makes it much easier to draw overall conclusions. Table 12.2 gives a hypothetical example of the assessment of an RCT. (Note: this is only an illustration, and only some of the critical and important causes of bias are listed.)

When assessing bias, a distinction needs to be made between critical and important causes of bias. In general, critical sources of bias equate to high risk and those that are important are classed as moderate risk. This approach was followed in Table 12.2. Sometimes an important cause of bias can lead to a rating of high risk. Consider the issue of imbalance at baseline in an RCT. Inadequate adjustment for this would usually be rated a moderate risk of bias. However, if the imbalance occurred in factors that were likely to influence the outcome (such as disease severity), and it was large enough to lead to substantial bias, the bias rating would be high.

Derive an overall rating

When the sources of bias and their effects have been listed, the overall risk of bias is commonly given a score on a three-point scale from low to high. The initial rating of the research design (Table 12.1) is

TABLE 12.2   Illustration of an assessment of risk of bias in an RCT.

Possible source of bias	Assessment	Risk of bias
Critical questions		
Method of randomisation	The randomisation was carried out by an independent clinical trials unit	Low
Loss to follow-up	Small difference: loss of 5% in control group and 10% in intervention group	Low
Selective reporting of outcomes	The primary outcome stated in the protocol was not mentioned in the published paper	High
Important questions		
Trial registration	No mention of trial registration	Moderate
The two groups are not comparable at baseline on one factor	The difference at baseline was small, with no obvious mechanism by which the factor would affect the outcome	Low
The measurement of the outcome	The outcome involved a subjective assessment of patient wellbeing. No mention was made of the training of the researchers who collected the data, nor of whether they were blind to treatment group	Moderate

modified according to the number of critical and moderate risks of bias. It is increased by two levels for each rating of high risk of bias. It is also increased by one level if there are two or more moderate risks of bias.

This system can be applied to the example in Table 12.2. An RCT design initially has a low level of bias, but the presence of one high risk of bias score increases the overall rating by two levels to become high. The addition of two moderate risk of bias scores leads to a further increase to make the final overall rating very high. Although the study has low ratings on the other risk of bias questions, these do not influence the overall score: good features do not compensate for serious flaws.

An advantage of this formal system is that it encourages a consistent approach to the evaluation of risk of bias. These rules are arbitrary, and individual researchers could modify them. For example, a new rule could be added that four or more important flaws could increase the risk of bias rating by two levels. However, adding complication increases the opportunities for mistakes; it is usually better to keep things simple.

Summary

A study's risk of bias depends on the research design and the nature and the number of the sources of bias. The initial level reflects the bias inherent in the research design. This is modified by the number of sources of moderate and high risk of bias to create an overall risk of bias score. This chapter has focused on the risk of bias of individual studies. Single studies can generate interesting findings, but they are much less convincing than systematic reviews of all relevant studies. Chapter 13 describes a method for assessing the certainty of evidence provided by systematic reviews.

CHAPTER 13

Certainty of Evidence

The concept of certainty of evidence was developed by the GRADE Working Group (Grading of Recommendations Assessment, Development and Evaluation). This is an international network of clinicians and researchers who have developed 'a common, sensible and transparent approach to grading quality (or certainty) of evidence and strength of recommendations' (https://www.gradeworkinggroup.org). This chapter reviews the nature of certainty of evidence, the factors that affect it, and how an overall assessment can be derived.

The nature of certainty of evidence

Certainty of evidence, sometimes termed quality of evidence, assesses the level of confidence in estimates of treatment effect. It is based on the findings from systematic reviews. Individual studies, even those of high quality, seldom provide convincing evidence. Tens of thousands of randomised controlled trials (RCTs) are published each year so, by chance alone, some of them will have misleading

The Pocket Guide to Critical Appraisal, Second Edition. Iain K. Crombie.
© 2022 John Wiley & Sons Ltd. Published 2022 by John Wiley & Sons Ltd.

large effect sizes. High-quality systematic reviews of RCTs provide strong evidence because they combine the results from several trials, reducing the impact of the play of chance.

An important contribution of the GRADE system is to emphasise that each of the outcomes presented in a systematic review should be assessed separately. Previously the overall quality of a systematic review was assessed, but the new approach recognises that when there are multiple outcomes these may differ in the quality of the evidence they provide.

The GRADE approach to certainty compares the observed effect size against a specified minimum benefit of a treatment. This is the amount of health benefit that would be needed to make the treatment clinically worthwhile. Certainty refers to the likelihood that the estimate of treatment effect is greater than this minimum benefit. It is rated on a four-point scale in which the highest level of certainty corresponds to 'very likely to exceed the specified minimum benefit', followed by 'likely to exceed it', 'unlikely to exceed it', with the lowest rating of 'very unlikely to do so'.

The first step of the GRADE process is to rate the certainty of evidence from systematic reviews of RCTs as high. Then it identifies two groups of factors, one that can downgrade certainty and one that can increase it. The next two sections describe these factors.

Downgrading the certainty of evidence

GRADE identifies five factors that can reduce confidence in the findings from a systematic review. The first is the risk of bias of the studies included in the review. The next three factors correspond to the value questions that were described in Chapter 5 of this book: imprecision, inconsistency, and indirectness. The last is publication bias, a potential weakness of systematic reviews. Deficiencies in any of the five factors will downgrade the certainty of evidence. It is reduced by one level if the flaw is serious, and two levels for very serious.

Risk of bias

The GRADE approach to assessing the risk of bias of RCTs included in a systematic review emphasises the need for a simple and parsimonious evaluation. It assesses five features of each RCT: allocation concealment, lack of blinding, loss to follow-up, deviation from intention to treat, and selective outcome reporting. (To simplify the assessment of bias, factors such as pre-registration of trials, adequacy of measurement of the outcomes, and conflicts of interest among the trial authors are not included.)

GRADE does not provide a method for summarising the bias of individual studies but recommends that the authors of the review make a judgement based on their evaluation of a trial. The method of summarising risk of bias described in Chapter 12 of this book provides a framework within which these judgements can be made.

Imprecision

Precision refers to the width of the confidence interval for the estimated treatment effect from a systematic review. The narrower the confidence interval, the greater the precision. Imprecision occurs when the confidence interval covers a wide range. For example, an interval that ranged from a very small to very large benefit would be judged imprecise. If the interval extended from possibly harmful to moderately beneficial, imprecision would be a serious concern.

Systematic reviews based on a few small RCTs present a challenge for the interpretation of precision. They raise the question of whether the included trials provide sufficient numbers of patients in total to provide reliable estimates of the confidence interval. As a rough guide, the total number of patients should be greater than 2000 and preferably more than 4000. A more formal approach is to determine what is known as the optimal information size (OIS): the minimum amount of information required to obtain reliable estimates from a systematic review. The calculation is similar to that used to obtain the required sample size for an RCT. In essence, it specifies the minimum clinically worthwhile effect, and then calculates the sample size needed to detect that effect size as being statistically significant. This calculated sample size is the OIS. If the total number of patients in the systematic review is bigger than the OIS, the precision is adequate. If it is lower than the OIS, the certainty of evidence is downgraded.

Inconsistency

The term inconsistency is the same as heterogeneity and was reviewed in Chapter 11. When some trials indicate that the treatment is effective, but others suggest the opposite, there is doubt about the meaning of the findings. This suspicion is increased if there is little overlap in the confidence intervals of the individual studies. Possible causes of heterogeneity should be explored, and statistical methods should be used to adjust for it. When lack of consistency across the component trials is not explored and explained, the certainty of the evidence is reduced.

Indirectness

The indirectness of a research finding is assessed by three factors, which were addressed by the questions of value in Chapter 5. These are: the importance of the outcome measure to patients, whether the characteristics of those on whom the intervention was tested are similar to those who would receive it in local clinical practice, and the availability of appropriate facilities and clinical expertise to support its use. Information on these topics is often limited in published systematic reviews. More detail might be obtained from the protocols and published papers of the studies included in the systematic reviews, although this may not always be sufficient to make a valid assessment. This limitation may make it difficult to conduct an informed assessment of indirectness.

Another type of indirectness occurs when the interest lies in comparing drug A against drug B. Sometimes there will be no trials that have conducted head-to-head evaluations of A against B. But when several studies have compared A against a placebo and others have assessed B against placebo, a statistical method (network meta-analysis) can be used to compare the effectiveness of A against that of B. The method assumes that the two groups of studies are similar in methodological quality, in the characteristics of patients recruited, the ancillary care received, and the measurement of the outcomes. This type of evidence is indirect because the assumptions of network meta-analysis may not be met.

Publication bias

Publication bias occurs when some of the trials of an intervention are not included in a systematic review. The results of some trials may not appear in medical journals because the researchers thought the findings were not interesting and decided not to publish them. Another reason is that journals may reject studies that they judge not worthy of publication. In addition, many systematic reviews restrict their searches to English-language journals, so that those studies written in other languages will be excluded. Finally, some studies only appear as abstracts in conference proceedings or in theses stored by universities and will often be overlooked.

A common finding is that unpublished and difficult-to-find studies often have small and non-statistically significant findings. Sometimes there is a delay of many years before studies with null findings are published. When some studies are not included in systematic reviews because of non-publication or delayed publication, the pooled effect size often overestimates the true value. Systematic reviews should carefully evaluate the extent and possible consequences of publication bias, through funnel plots and statistical methods. Inadequate investigation of this issue means the pooled effect size could be biased and the certainty of evidence is downgraded.

Factors that increase certainty

Three of the questions about value may increase the rating of certainty. These are: large effect size, dose–response effect, and the possible impact of unmeasured or residual confounding. If the study scores well on one of these items, it can be moved up one level, although it cannot attain a higher level than that originally assigned to the systematic review.

Large effect size

A large effect size can provide protection against bias. Most causes of bias have, on average, only a modest impact on effect size. Thus, a large relative risk of ≥ 5.0 is unlikely to be solely due to bias. Evidence that has been downgraded because of bias may be upgraded if the effect size is large. This type of moderation should be made with care, as it is possible that, in a particular instance, the impact of bias was much larger than the average.

Dose–response gradient

A dose–response effect occurs when the frequency of an outcome increases (or decreases) with the amount of treatment given. A simple example is a trial of a new drug where patients were randomised to one of three groups: control group, low-dose group, and high-dose group. If the low dose had a better outcome than the control group and the high dose was better still, there is a dose–response effect. The benefit of a dose–response relationship is that it is unlikely to be caused by bias. It is difficult to see how factors such as concealment of treatment allocation could vary systematically with the amount of drug administered to produce a dose–response effect.

Effect of unmeasured or residual confounding factors

Cohort and case-control studies are considered at high risk of bias because of concerns about unmeasured confounding factors. Because they cannot be measured, these confounding factors may lead to overestimates of the true effect sizes. Cohort and case-control studies are given a high bias rating because of the possibility that there is an inability to adjust for the unmeasured confounding.

Although confounding factors usually increase the observed (unadjusted) effect size, they may sometimes have the opposite effect of reducing the effect size. In that case, if adjustment was made for the confounding, the effect size would be increased. This is sometimes called reverse confounding. It would seem unreasonable to assign a high risk of bias to cohort and case–control studies in circumstances when the unmeasured confounders are likely to have reduced the observed effect size. This argument for increasing the certainty of evidence relies on knowing all the unmeasured confounders and being sure how they will influence the effect size. Such circumstances will not be common and the upgrading will rarely happen.

Overall assessment of certainty

To obtain an overall assessment of certainty GRADE rates a systematic review of RCTs as high. Then each of the five factors for downgrading is given a score to reflect its weaknesses: −1 for serious concerns and −2 if concerns are very serious. Similarly, the factors for upgrading are given a score of +1 if they meet the criteria for mitigation (with the exception that effect size is scored +1 for large effect and +2 for very large).

This method could suggest that an overall score could be calculated by adding up the scores. GRADE advises against this mechanistic approach to assessing certainty. It recommends that judgement is used to evaluate the impact of the factors on the certainty of evidence, with the individual scores providing a basis for making a considered decision. Caution should be used in rating up certainty of evidence, as the circumstances in which this is justified will rarely occur. It would only be justified when limitations have resulted in downgrading, and there is a convincing case for increasing certainty of evidence.

Conclusion

This chapter has explored how the findings from critical appraisal can be synthesised to draw conclusions about the certainty of evidence. Each of the outcomes of a systematic review is rated on a four-point scale from 'likely to exceed a threshold for a minimum benefit of a treatment' to 'very unlikely to do so'. This rating is determined by five factors that can downgrade certainty and three that can upgrade it. In producing this framework for making and reporting decisions in a transparent manner, the GRADE collaboration has made a major contribution to assessing research evidence. The concept of certainty of evidence is a substantial advance on the previous approach, which relied on the effect size and its confidence interval. The focus on assessing individual outcomes separately is another important feature of GRADE.

GRADE also emphasises that certainty evidence is not the only factor that determines recommendations for clinical practice. Making decisions about which treatments should be used involves other considerations that relate to value, such as the benefit to harm ratio, cost, and health equity (issues of fairness and impact on inequalities in health). These issues are discussed in Chapter 14.

CHAPTER 14

Assessing Value

This book has focused on assessing value based on the results of research studies published in medical journals. The key issues are the clinical importance of the findings (effect size, precision, and consistency with previous research), their relevance to patients, and their suitability for the local health care system. Published papers should provide sufficient information to enable a critical appraisal of these issues, although sometimes the information provided will be limited.

Professional groups concerned with funding, managing, and delivering health care have to assess many aspects of value in addition to effect size and precision. The cost of treatments is a key concern. All healthcare systems strive to provide high-quality care, but do so within fixed budgets. Even the wealthiest of countries have struggled to cope with the continuous rise in the cost of health care. This has focused attention on achieving the maximum value from the available resources. The net health benefit is determined by the effectiveness of individual treatments, their potential for harm, and the benefit to harm ratio. This can be compared with the cost of

The Pocket Guide to Critical Appraisal, Second Edition. Iain K. Crombie.
© 2022 John Wiley & Sons Ltd. Published 2022 by John Wiley & Sons Ltd.

the treatment to ensure the greatest health gain from the funding available.

More recently other issues have been identified as important, such as the extent of unmet need and the broader societal concerns with health equity. The principles of social justice hold that the delivery of health care should be fair and compassionate, respecting individual rights, treating patients with dignity, and safeguarding the vulnerable. Value is now regarded as a much broader concept than benefit, harm, and cost. Health care should provide timely access to appropriate treatment for all according to their need.

Many national and international organisations have developed methods for assessing value to facilitate the setting of priorities and the allocation of resources within health care systems (see the Appendix: Further Reading). The common aim is to provide a framework for assessing the value of treatments to identify those that should be prioritised by health care systems. Although there are some differences in the approaches taken, there is substantial agreement on the main components of value.

This chapter gives a brief introduction to the important components of value. These are organised under five headings covering benefits, harms, costs, feasibility, and health equity. This chapter also shows how the value questions from Chapter 5 are incorporated into this broader framework and identifies many of the challenges in measuring the components of value.

Measuring potential benefit

In previous chapters the benefit of a treatment has focused on the findings of research studies on groups of patients. However, from a societal perspective the interest lies in the health gain that will be achieved when the treatment is rolled out across the whole population. To assess this broader view of benefit three additional factors need to be considered.

The burden of the disease

The value of an intervention also depends on the nature of the disease being treated. The more common it is and the greater the amount of suffering caused, the higher is the potential benefit from treatment. Thus information is needed on the number of new cases that will occur each year and the impact the disease has on length and quality of life. Another key issue is the extent of unmet need given current health care provision. If other treatments are available to treat a disease, then value depends on how much additional benefit the new treatment provides. The focus is on the net gain to society.

Duration of benefit

Some interventions, such as immunisation against measles, can provide lifelong protection. However, some diseases, such as depression, spontaneous pneumothorax, or hydatid cyst of the liver, can recur after treatment. Their benefit will depend on the average duration of the disease-free interval. As most clinical trials have only a short time frame, they may overestimate the true benefit of a treatment.

Timely delivery

In many clinical situations the best outcomes will be achieved by timely delivery of care. Examples include the treatment of heart attacks and the diagnosis and management of cancer. When tested in research studies, efforts are made to ensure that treatments are delivered promptly. This may not be possible in routine care for busy health professionals who have to cope with many demands on their time. Care is needed when assessing the likely benefit of a treatment that works best when delivered promptly.

Harm and the balance between benefit and harm

Measuring harms

Many treatments cause side effects and, although these are usually minor, serious adverse effects do occur. Obtaining data on the severity and frequency of harms is challenging. Randomised controlled trials (RCTs) commonly have modest numbers of participants and short follow-up periods, so rare and long-term adverse events will not be detected. Trials frequently underreport the adverse events that are detected and often only state the total number of patients who experience adverse events, so that information on severity is not available. When data on individual harms are presented, there is often a lack of consistency in the definitions (diagnostic criteria) that are used, making it difficult to estimate an average across studies. Systematic reviews often do not mention adverse events reported in RCTs. Finally, the patient perspective on harms is seldom assessed.

The difficulty of measuring harms has been recognised by national and international regulatory authorities. These bodies are responsible for ensuring the efficacy and safety of medicines. They have launched initiatives to develop methods and procedures for assessing harm. Pharmacoepidemiology studies that assess the effects of drugs as they are used in clinical practice can help identify rare and long-term harms. These can be large cohort studies, or case–control studies, designed specifically to detect adverse events. Accessing this evidence may require searching for recent systematic reviews of such studies or conducting a new systematic review. For many treatments few pharmacoepidemiology studies will be available, although this should improve with the new initiatives underway.

The balance between benefit and harm

The value of a treatment will depend on the balance between the magnitude of the benefit and the frequency and severity of the harm. Considerable effort is made to estimate treatment benefit accurately, to assess its precision, and to evaluate bias. By contrast, the measurement of harm receives much less attention. The limited and potentially unreliable evidence on adverse effects makes it difficult to derive benefit to harm ratios. As harms are often underreported, these ratios may be biased in favour of benefits.

Costs and cost effectiveness

As resources for health are limited, cost is central to decisions about the value of a treatment. For example, an expensive treatment would have to provide substantial benefit to be used in clinical practice, whereas a more modestly priced treatment with a smaller benefit might be recommended. In health economics value is measured as the patient benefit compared to the cost of treatment. Two types of cost are recognised: direct and indirect. The direct costs include the medication, the health care staff, the use of equipment and premises, and the administrative costs of running the health care centre. The indirect costs are those that result from the illness, such as loss of income, reduced economic productivity, and the intangible costs of pain and suffering.

A widely used method to balance benefit and expenditure is cost effectiveness analysis (CEA). It measures the benefit by estimating the number of extra years of life that will be lived, adjusting this for any impairment in the quality of life. This is expressed as a QALY (Quality Adjusted Life Years), where one year of life in perfect health is one QALY. For example, a treatment that added five extra years of life at only 60% of the maximum possible quality would generate 3 QALYs (5×0.6). If that treatment cost £30 000, it would have a cost per QALY of £10 000 (£30 000 ÷ 3). The cost per QALY provides a convenient measure to compare the cost effectiveness of treatments. The calculation requires good data on the components of costs and on the quality of life following treatment.

Opportunity cost

A consequence of fixed health care budgets is that new interventions, particularly expensive ones, can only be implemented by reducing investment in another existing treatment or service. This creates what is called opportunity cost – the amount of health benefit lost by disinvesting in some types of care. The result is that the net benefit of a new intervention will be the number of QALYs it provides minus the QALYs from the treatment that was displaced.

Feasibility of implementation of a treatment

Suitability for a health care system

The feasibility of implementing a new intervention will depend on the technical challenges of delivering it and the capacity of the health care system to deliver it. These include the availability of skilled staff, and their willingness to adopt a new therapy or diagnostic tool. It will also need the appropriate infrastructure to support intervention delivery, such as the premises, diagnostic and other equipment, information technology, and administrative support. To ensure coherent delivery of care, the new procedure should be co-located with related services. Implementation may be difficult for treatments that require sophisticated diagnostic facilities, intensive monitoring, or extended stays in hospital.

Acceptability to patients and carers

Any new intervention should be acceptable to patients and their carers. This is important on moral grounds, but will also affect the uptake and the health gain from specific treatments. For patients, factors that reduce acceptability could include the impositions that treatment involves such as fasting prior to attendance, the inconvenience of in-patient stays, and pain and discomfort during treatment and in the recovery period. Compared with evidence on the effectiveness of treatments, there are few studies on acceptability.

Health equity

The World Health Organization emphasises that attaining the highest possible standard of health is a basic human right. Health inequity occurs when some groups or individuals experience poor health outcomes that could have been prevented or treated. The fair innings argument holds that health care resources should be distributed so that everyone has the opportunity to live for the normal span of years in reasonably good health. Health equity depends on the accessibility of treatments and the fair and compassionate delivery of care.

Accessibility

Accessibility refers to the ease with which patients can access a health care service. The inverse care law describes the challenge: those most in need of treatment can be least likely to receive it. Issues such as lack of transport, difficulty of taking time off work, or concerns about cost can act as barriers to access. Lack of knowledge about the benefits of an intervention may deter health care seeking. Well-educated, affluent individuals are more likely to know about and to request new treatments.

The accessibility of health care will vary across groups and regions of a country. Small towns and rural communities will often have reduced access to specialist services with sophisticated equipment. Socially disadvantaged groups often face more difficulties in accessing care. In the case of mental health, concerns about stigma may deter attendance at clinics.

To ensure that difficulties of access to a treatment do not cause health inequity, additional support can be directed to disadvantaged or vulnerable groups. This would provide information about the treatment options and enable access to appropriate care. Such action would increase the cost per QALY. Societies have to decide how much extra they are prepared to spend to ensure that everyone receives timely treatment according to their need.

The worse-off principle

The principle of equal treatment for all may be deliberately broken in some circumstances. For example, a higher value may be given to a treatment for a severe disease if it will make a substantial difference to length or quality of life. This is called the worse-off principle in which treatments for severe diseases are accorded a higher value than those for less serious illnesses. Alleviating suffering among those who are severely ill is justified by the argument that, where possible, everyone should have a basic minimum quality of life, sufficient 'to make a life worth living'. This can justify a higher cost per QALY for treating diseases that substantially diminish quality of life.

A particular case of the worse-off principle concerns individuals who are in immediate risk of dying or sustaining serious injury. This has been termed the rule of rescue, in which events such as traffic accidents, heart attacks, or violent assaults are given special priority. Few would argue that treatment for these events should only be given if this was justified by the cost per QALY.

Special attention is also given to those with a terminal illness, where a few months of additional life could be highly valued. The case for prioritising young children with serious or life-threatening illness is even stronger. As they have enjoyed so few years of life, it would seem fair to spend a little extra to relieve their symptoms and extend their lives. Cost effectiveness may have to take second place when there are considerations of fairness, urgency, and the duty to save lives.

Summary

This chapter has reviewed the range of issues that determine the value of treatments. These include cost effectiveness, benefit to harm ratios, the clinical context, the nature of the local health care system, and societal views on health equity.

The task of assessing value is commonly undertaken by multi-disciplinary teams comprising clinicians, health economists, health service researchers, health care administrators, and policy makers, supported by information specialists who search for evidence to support decision making. These teams have the resources to collect additional information, and the wide range of expertise needed to make informed assessments of feasibility, cost, benefit, and equity.

To ensure fairness, the process should be systematic, objective, and transparent.

Balancing the many complex issues that comprise value is difficult. Some of the topics, such as cost and health equity, are measured on different scales making them difficult to compare. For others, such as harms, patient preferences, and feasibility of implementation, the available information may be limited. Further, many of the decisions require subjective judgements, so that even reasonable people might disagree on the setting of priorities.

A common approach is to assess the components of value then use judgement to derive an overall rating for each treatment. This could be supported by the technique of multi-criteria decision analysis (MCDA), which proposes that each component (criterion) is assigned a numerical weight (such as zero, one, or two) to reflect its perceived importance. Acting individually, members of the assessment committee could assign scores to each component and then, by discussion and debate, arrive at a consensus.

The method of MCDA can combine the scores in a mathematical model to derive a total score for each treatment. This type of calculation is not widely favoured. A weakness is that poor performance on one criterion could be overwhelmed by the scores on the other criteria. This might not be helpful if, for example, feasibility of implementation had a low score but the total score was high. It would seem unwise to recommend a treatment that could not easily be implemented.

In conclusion, the value of treatments is assessed by a diverse array of criteria. At present there is not a universally agreed definition of value, although there is broad consensus about its main components. The main challenges are the limited evidence available for the assessment of some criteria and the lack of an agreed method for deriving an overall score. Despite these difficulties, decisions about resource allocation have to be made. The current components of value provide a more acceptable and defensible approach than an exclusive focus on cost effectiveness.

Appendix: Further Reading

This Appendix presents papers, reports, and websites that expand on the ideas and topics covered in this book. Much of the literature on medical research is highly technical so only sources that are readily accessible are listed. Several authoritative bodies have constructed sets of critical appraisal tools, which are available from their websites. To avoid repetition these are listed in Chapter 1 and are not repeated in the further reading for Chapters 6–11. Additional sources of appraisal tools for individual research designs are listed in the appropriate chapters when these could be helpful.

Chapter 1: Introduction

1. Sets of critical appraisal tools, covering the main research designs, are available from several websites (see the text that follows). The websites differ in the range of research designs covered. The tools for individual designs vary in length and content, and the questions for specific issues are often phrased differently. Most provide helpful explanations for the items included:
   - The Critical Appraisal Skills Programme (CASP) https://casp-uk.net/casp-tools-checklists/.
   - The Joanna Brigs Institute (JBI) https://joannabriggs.org/critical-appraisal-tools.

The Pocket Guide to Critical Appraisal, Second Edition. Iain K. Crombie.
© 2022 John Wiley & Sons Ltd. Published 2022 by John Wiley & Sons Ltd.

- The Centre for Evidence-Based Medicine `https://www.cebm.ox.ac.uk/resources/ebm-tools/critical-appraisal-tools`.
- Scottish Intercollegiate Network Guidelines (SIGN) `https://www.sign.ac.uk/what-we-do/methodology/checklists/`.
- The National Institute for Health and Care Excellence (NICE) `https://www.nice.org.uk/process/pmg6/resources/the-guidelines-manual-appendices-bi-2549703709/chapter/appendix-b-methodology-checklist-systematic-reviews-and-meta-analyses`.
- The US National Institutes of Health (NIH) and the National Heart, Lung and Blood Institute `https://www.nhlbi.nih.gov/health-topics/study-quality-assessment-tools`.
- BMJ tools `https://bestpractice.bmj.com/info/toolkit/ebm-toolbox/critical-appraisal-checklists/`.

2. Lucid accounts of many of the important ideas in critical appraisal are presented in these three papers:
   - Burls A. *What Is Critical Appraisal?* 2nd edn. Oxford, UK: University of Oxford, 2009. `https://citeseerx.ist.psu.edu/viewdoc/download?doi=10.1.1.734.5910&rep=rep1&type=pdf` (accessed 28 January 2021).
   - Jackson R, Maeratunga S, Broad J et al. The GATE frame: critical appraisal with pictures. *EBM* 2006; 11: 35–38.
   - Young JM, Solomon MJ. How to critically appraise an article. *Nature Clinical Practice Gastroenterol Hepatol* 2009; 6: 82–91.

3. Several research groups have systematically identified and reviewed the contents of individual critical appraisals tools. The findings are that these tools vary in quality and content, although the tools for clinical trials are often of higher quality than those for other research designs. For many research

designs some important issues are poorly addressed. Some illustrative studies are listed in the text that follows:

- Crowe M, Sheppard L. A review of critical appraisal tools show they lack rigor: alternative tool structure is proposed. *J Clin Epidemiol* 2011, 64: 79–80. https://doi.org/10.1016/j.jclinepi.2010.02.008.
- Lundh A, Rasmussen K, Ostengaard L et al. Systematic review finds that appraisal tools for medical research studies address conflicts of interest superficially. *J Clin Epidemiol* 2020; 120: 104–115. https://doi.org/10.1016/j.jclinepi.2019.12.005.
- Zeng X, Zhang Y, Kwong JSW et al. The methodological quality assessment tools for preclinical and clinical studies, systematic review and meta-analysis, and clinical practice guideline: a systematic review. *J Evid Based Med* 2015; 8: 2–10, doi: 10.1111/jebm.1214.
- Page MJ, McKenzie JE, Higgins JPT. Tools for assessing risk of reporting biases in studies and syntheses of studies: a systematic review. *BMJ Open* 2018; 8: e019703. doi: 10.1136/bmjopen-2017-019703.
- Sanderson S, Tatt ID, Higgins JPT. Tools for assessing quality and susceptibility to bias in observational studies in epidemiology: a systematic review and annotated bibliography. *Int J Epidemiol* 2007; 36: 666–676. https://doi.org/10.1093/ije/dym018.

Chapter 3: Identifying the research design

1. A website created by the Centre for Evidence Based Medicine at the University of Oxford gives a brief outline of the main study designs: https://www.cebm.ox.ac.uk/resources/ebm-tools/study-designs.
2. Helpful guidance on the identification of research designs is given in these two papers:
   - Sut N. Study designs in medicine. *Balkan Med J* 2014, 4; 273–277. doi: 10.5152/balkanmedj.2014.1408.

- Chidambaram AG, Josephson M. Clinical research study designs: the essentials. *Pediatric Invest* 2019; 4: 245–252. https://doi.org/10.1002/ped4.12166.

Chapter 4: Interpreting the results

1. Several measures of effect sizes are described in this informative paper:
   - Tripepi G, Jager KJ, Dekker FW et al. Measures of effect: relative risks, odds ratios, risk difference, and 'number needed to treat'. *Kidney Internat* 2007; 72: 789–791. https://doi.org/10.1038/sj.ki.5002432.

2. Significance testing and p-values are frequently misused. These four papers outline the common misunderstandings of these statistical procedures, and the ways that they are abused:
   - Gagnier JJ, Morgenstern H. Misconceptions, misuses, and misinterpretations of p values and significance testing. *J Bone Joint Surg Am* 2017; 99: 1598–1603.
   - Mills JL. Data torturing. *N Engl J Med* 1993; 329: 1196–1199.
   - Wasserstein RL, Lazar NA. The ASA's statement on p-values: context, process, and purpose. *Am Statist* 2016; 70: 129–131.
   - Goodman SN. Toward evidence-based medical statistics. 1: The p value fallacy. *Ann Intern Med* 1999; 130: 995–1004.

3. This website, created by CEBM at the University of Oxford, presents a catalogue of biases. It gives an explanation of each bias with examples to show how it can occur:
   - https://catalogofbias.org/.

4. Helpful explanations of the biases that afflict medical research are given in these three papers:
   - Delgado-Rodriguez M, Llorca J. Bias. *J Epidemiol Community Health* 2004; 58: 635–641. doi: 10.1136/jech.2003.008466.
   - Hartman JM, Forsen JW, Wallace MS et al. Tutorials in clinical research: Part IV: Recognizing and controlling bias. *Laringoscope* 2002; 112: 23–31.

- Pinar AY. Bias in epidemiological studies: a special focus on pediatric research. *J Pediatric Sci* 2009; 1: e9.

5. Confounding is a major problem for most research designs. The first two of the following five papers help clarify what confounding is and the next three papers describe the methods that are used to control for it:

   - Jager KJ, Zoccali C, McLeod A et al. Confounding: what it is and how to deal with it. *Kidney Internat* 2008; 73: 256–260. https://doi.org/10.1038/sj.ki.5002650.

   - Kyriacou N, Lewis RJ. Confounding by indication in clinical research. *JAMA* 2016, 17; 1818–1819. doi: 10.1001/jama.2016.16435.

   - Yu LM, Chan AW, Hopewell S et al. Reporting on covariate adjustment in randomised controlled trials before and after revision of the 2001 CONSORT statement: a literature review. *Trials* 2010, 11; 59. doi: 10.1186/1745-6215-11-59.

   - Kahan BC, Jairath V, Dore CJ et al. The risks and rewards of covariate adjustment in randomized trials: an assessment of 12 outcomes from 8 studies. *Trials* 2014, 15; 139. doi: 10.1186/1745-6215-15-139.

   - Raab GM, Day S, Sales J. How to select covariates to include in the analysis of a clinical trial. *Control Clin Trials* 2000; 21: 330–342.

6. The statistical analysis of research studies is sometimes manipulated. Chapter 4 of this book describes some of the techniques that may be used to distort the findings:

   - Crombie IK. Can the analysis bias the findings? *Evidence in Medicine: The Flaws, Their Causes and How to Prevent Them.* pp. 64–80. Chichester, UK: John Wiley and Sons, 2021.

Chapter 5: The in-depth interrogation

1. Many of the important issues in critical appraisal are covered in the second half of a chapter from a textbook on evidence-based medicine. The chapter is available online:

- Twells LK. Evidence-based decision-making 1: critical appraisal. In PS Parfrey and BJ Barrett (eds), *Clinical Epidemiology: Practice and Methods*, Methods in Molecular Biology, vol. 1281, pp. 385–395. New York: Springer Science+Business Media, 2015. doi: 10.1007/978-1-4939-2428-8_23.

2. This book makes the important distinction between risk of bias and the issues that are relevant for assessing value. Although it focuses on systematic reviews, the conceptual approach is relevant for all other quantitative research designs. It is available online:
   - Viswanathan M, Patnode CD, Berkman ND et al. *Methods Guide for Effectiveness and Comparative Effectiveness Reviews*. Rockville, MD: Agency for Healthcare Research and Quality, 2017. Available from: https://www.ncbi .nlm.nih.gov/sites/books/NBK519366/ (accessed 9 February 2021).

3. This paper presents a set of general questions for critical appraisal and gives useful descriptions of the issues that underlie these questions:
   - Al-Jundi A, Sakka S. Critical appraisal of clinical research. *J Clin Diag Res* 2017; 11(5): JE01–JE05. doi: 10.7860/JCDR/2017/26047.9942.

4. Research funded by the pharmaceutical industry can raise issues of conflict of interest (these companies will make substantial profits if randomised controlled trials [RCTs] show their products are effective). This paper cites several detailed reviews which highlight the distorting effect that industry studies can have on medical evidence:

   Moynihan R, Bero L, Hill S et al. Pathways to independence: towards producing and using trustworthy evidence. *BMJ* 2019; 367. https://doi.org/10.1136/ bmj.l6576.

Chapter 6: Appraising surveys

1. Of all the research designs, surveys are usually considered the easiest to carry out. In practice many surveys are poorly conducted. These four papers review the important issues for the design, conduct and interpretation of surveys:

   - Kelley K, Clark B, Brown V et al. Good practice in the conduct and reporting of survey research. *Int J Qual Health Care* 2005; 15: 262–266. https://doi.org/10.1093/intqhc/mzg031.

   - Draugalis JL, Coons SJ, Plaza CM. Best Practices for survey research reports: a synopsis for authors and reviewers. *Am J Pharmac Educ* 2008; 72: 11. https://doi.org/10.5688/aj720111.

   - Rybakov KN, Beckett R, Dilley I et al. Reporting quality of survey research articles published in the pharmacy literature. *Res Soc Admin Pharm* 2020, 16; 1354–1358. https://doi.org/10.1016/j.sapharm.2020.01.005.

   - Levin KA. Study design III: Cross-sectional studies. *Evid Based Dent* 2006; 7: 24–25. doi: 10.1038/sj.ebd.6400375.

2. Useful guidance for the critical appraisal of surveys is presented in these two papers:

   - Downes MJ, Brennan ML, Williams HC et al. Development of a critical appraisal tool to assess the quality of cross-sectional studies (AXIS). *BMJ Open* 2016; 6: e011458. doi: 10.1136/bmjopen-2016-011458.

   - Burns KEA, Kho ME. How to assess a survey report: a guide for readers and peer reviewers. *CMAJ* 2015; 187: E198–E205. doi: 10.1503/cmaj.140545.

Chapter 7: Appraising cohort studies

1. The main features of the design of cohort studies are reviewed in these three papers:
   - Caruana EJ, Roman M, Hernandez-Sanchez J et al. Longitudinal studies. *J Thorac Dis* 2015 Nov; 7(11): E537–E540. doi: 10.3978/j.issn.2072-1439.2015.10.63.
   - Grimes DA, Schultz KF. Cohort studies: marching towards outcomes. *Lancet* 2002; 359: 341–345. https://doi.org/10.1016/S0140-6736(02)07500-1.
   - Levin KA. Study design IV. Cohort studies. *Evid Based Dent* 2003; 7: 51–52. doi: 10.1038/sj.ebd.6400407.
2. Important issues for the critical appraisal of cohort studies are covered in these three papers:
   - Rochon PA, Gurwitz JH, Sykora K et al. Reader's guide to critical appraisal of cohort studies: role and design. *BMJ* 2005; 330: 895–897.
   - Mandani M, Sykora K, Li P et al. Reader's guide to critical appraisal of cohort studies: 2. Assessing potential for confounding. *BMJ* 2005; 330: 960–962. https://doi.org/10.1136/bmj.330.7497.960.
   - Normand S-L, Sykora K, Li P et al. Readers guide to critical appraisal of cohort studies: 3. Analytical strategies to reduce confounding. *BMJ* 2005; 330: 1021–1023. https://doi.org/10.1136/bmj.330.7498.1021.

Chapter 8: Appraising case–control studies

1. The case–control study is more likely to suffer from bias than many other research designs. The challenges for this design and the biases that can occur are outlined in these two papers:
   - Schultz KF, Grimes DA. Case–control studies: research in reverse. *Lancet* 2002; 359: 431–434. https://doi.org/10.1016/S0140-6736(02)07605-5.

- Kopec JA, Esdaile JM. Bias in case–control studies. A review. *J Epidemiol Community Health* 1990; 44: 179–186.

2. The main elements of the design and conduct of case–control studies are clearly described in this book. There are more recent books on the topic, but these often focus on the statistical analysis, adopting a mathematical approach. The readability of Schlesselman's book outweighs the shortcomings of its age:

   - Schlesselman JJ. *Case–Control Studies: Design, Conduct and Analysis*. Oxford, UK: Oxford University Press, 1982.

Chapter 9: Appraising randomised controlled trials

1. Helpful explanations of the critical appraisal questions for RCTs are outlined in these two papers. They differ slightly in the items that are included, but both make many good points:

   - Godin K, Dhillon M, Bhandari M. The three-minute appraisal of a randomized trial. *Indian J Orthop* 2011; 45: 194–196.

   - Roever L, Oliveira GBF. Critical appraisal of randomised controlled trials. *Evid Based Med Pract* 2016; 2: 1. doi: 10.4172/2471-9919.1000e114.

2. This paper describes many of the biases that afflict RCTs:

   - Sedgwick P. Bias in experimental study designs: randomised controlled trials with parallel groups. *BMJ* 2015; 351: h3869. https://www.bmj.com/content/351/bmj.h3869.

3. RCTs are often poorly conducted. Chapters 2 and 3 of this book describe the common deficiencies in clinical trials and their consequences:

- Crombie IK. *Evidence in Medicine: The Flaws, Their Causes and How to Prevent Them.* Chichester, UK: John Wiley and Sons, 2021.

Chapter 10: Cohort studies that evaluate the effectiveness of interventions

1. The use of cohort studies to assess the effectiveness of treatments is a much-debated topic. These papers review the main issues:

   - Hampson G, Towse A, Dreitlin WB et al. Real-world evidence for coverage decisions: opportunities and challenges. *J Compar Effect Res* 2018; 7: 1133–1143.
   - Franklin JM, Schneeweiss S. When and how can real world data analyses substitute for randomized controlled trials? *Clin Pharmac Therapeut* 2017; 102: 924–933. doi: 10.1002/cpt.857.
   - Gerstein HC, McMurray J, Holman RR. Real-world studies no substitute for RCTs in establishing efficacy. *Lancet* 2019; 393: 210–211.

2. The critical appraisal of cohort studies that evaluate the effectiveness of interventions is challenging because of the complexity of many of the issues which need to be addressed. These papers give explanations of the key topics as well as guidance and specific prompts to lead to a judgement on the overall risk of bias:

   - Sterne JAC, Hernán MA, Reeves BC et al. ROBINS-I: a tool for assessing risk of bias in non-randomised studies of interventions. *BMJ* 2016; 355: i4919. https://doi.org/10.1136/bmj.i4919.
   - D'Endrea E, Vinals L, Patorno E et al. How well can we assess the validity of non-randomised studies of medications? A systematic review of assessment tools. *BMJ Open* 2021; 11: e043961. doi: 10.1136/bmjopen-2020-043961.

- Wells GA, Shea B, Higgins JPT et al. Checklists of methodological issues for review authors to consider when including non-randomized studies in systematic reviews. *Res Synth Meth* 2013; 4: 63–77. doi: 10.1002/jrsm.1077. https://onlinelibrary.wiley.com/doi/epdf/10.1002/jrsm.1077?saml_referrer.

- Quigley JM, Thompson JC, Halfpenny NJ et al. Critical appraisal of nonrandomized studies – a review of recommended and commonly used tools. *J Eval Clin Pract* 2019; 25: 44–52.

- Kim SY, Park JE, Lee YJ et al. Testing a tool for assessing the risk of bias for nonrandomized studies showed moderate reliability and promising validity. *J Clin Epidemiol* 2013; 66: 408–414. https://doi.org/10.1016/j.jclinepi.2012.09.016.

- Deeks JJ, Dinnes J, D'Amico R et al. Evaluating non-randomised intervention studies. *Health Technol Assess* 2003; 7: 27. https://www.journalslibrary.nihr.ac.uk/hta/hta7270/#/abstract.

- Coles B, Tyrer F, Hussein H et al. Development, content validation, and reliability of the Assessment of Real-World Observational Studies (ArRoWS) critical appraisal tool. *Ann Epidemiol* 2020; 55: 57–63.e15. https://doi.org/10.1016/j.annepidem.2020.09.014.

3. The tools used to evaluate the risk of bias in non-randomised studies often have limitations. These papers explore the weaknesses. The findings are directly relevant for cohort studies which evaluate the effectiveness of interventions:

   - Jeyaraman MM, Rabbani R, Copstein L et al. Methodologically rigorous risk of bias tools for nonrandomized studies had low reliability and high evaluator burden. *J Clin Epidemiol* 2020; 120: 140–147.

   - Kim SY, Park JE, Lee YJ et al. Testing a tool for assessing the risk of bias for nonrandomized studies showed moderate reliability and promising validity. *J Clin Epidemiol* 2013; 66: 408–414. https://doi.org/10.1016/j.jclinepi.2012.09.016.

Chapter 11: Appraising systematic reviews

1. The most authoritative text on the conduct, and the flaws, in systematic reviews is that produced by the Cochrane Collaboration. Their Handbook and the supportive materials on their website (www.cochrane.org) give well-written and thorough explanations of all aspects of this research design:
   - Higgins J, Thomas J, Chandler J et al., editors. *Cochrane Handbook for Systematic Reviews of Interventions*. 2nd ed. Chichester, UK: John Wiley & Sons, 2019.

2. Publication bias can be detected by the graphical technique, funnel plots. This paper describes a useful method for conducting and interpreting these plots:
   - Peters JL, Sutton AJ, Jones DR et al. Contour-enhanced meta-analysis funnel plots help distinguish publication bias from other causes of asymmetry. *J Clin Epidemiol* 2008; 61: 991–996.

3. Two tools, the AMSTAR (A MeaSurement Tool to Assess Systematic Reviews) tool and the ROBIS (Risk of Bias in Systematic Reviews) tool, are frequently used for the critical appraisal of systematic reviews. The following papers describe these tools:
   - Shea BJ, Grimshaw JM, Wells GA et al. Development of AMSTAR: a measurement tool to assess the methodological quality of systematic reviews. *BMC Med Res Methodol* 2007; 7: 10. https://doi.org/10.1186/1471-2288-7-10.
   - Shea BJ, Reeves BC, Wells GA et al. AMSTAR 2: a critical appraisal tool for systematic reviews that include randomised or non-randomised studies of healthcare interventions, or both. BMJ 2017; 358: j4008. doi: 10.1136/bmj.j40.
   - Faggion CM, Jr. Critical appraisal of AMSTAR: challenges, limitations, and potential solutions from the perspective of an assessor. *BMC Med Res Methodol* 2015; 15: 63. http://dx.doi.org/10.1186/s12874-015-0062-6.

- Whiting P, Savović J, Higgins JP et al. ROBIS: a new tool to assess risk of bias in systematic reviews was developed. *J Clin Epidemiol* 2016; 69(1): 225–234. http://dx.doi.org/10.1016/j.jclinepi.2015.06.005.

Chapter 12: Summarising risk of bias

Critical appraisal identifies the potential sources of bias in research studies but does not provide an overall estimate of the amount of bias in individual studies. Simply counting the number of biases is unhelpful because it assigns equal weight to each component. A book chapter and two papers provide more thoughtful approaches to summarising bias:

- Higgins J, Savović J, Page M et al. Assessing risk of bias in a randomized trial. In J Higgins, J Thomas, J Chandler et al., *Cochrane Handbook for Systematic Reviews of Interventions.* 2nd edn, pp. 205–228. Chichester, UK: John Wiley & Sons, 2019.
- Guyatt GH, Oxman AD, Vist G et al. GRADE guidelines: 4. Rating the quality of evidence – study limitations (risk of bias). *J Clin Epidemiol* 2011; 64: 407–415. doi: 10.1016/j.jclinepi.2010.07.017.
- Shea BJ, Reeves BC, Wells GA et al. AMSTAR 2: a critical appraisal tool for systematic reviews that include randomised or non-randomised studies of healthcare interventions, or both. *BMJ* 2017; 358: j4008. doi: 10.1136/bmj.j40.

Chapter 13: Certainty of evidence

1. The GRADE Working Group is an international collaboration of experts that has developed extensive guidance on the interpretation and evaluation of research evidence. The first four papers describe the components of certainty of evidence.

The final two papers outline the approach to synthesising the findings to derive an overall evaluation of certainty of evidence:

- Guyatt GH, Oxman AD, Montori V et al. GRADE guidelines: 5. Rating the quality of evidence – publication bias. *J Clin Epidemiol* 2011; 64: 1277–1282. doi: 10.1016/j.jclinepi .2011.01.011.
- Guyatt GH, Oxman AD, Kunz R et al. GRADE guidelines: 6. Rating the quality of evidence – imprecision. *J Clin Epidemiol* 2011; 64: 1283–1293. doi: 10.1016/j.jclinepi .2011.01.012.
- Guyatt GH, Oxman AD, Kunz R et al. GRADE guidelines: 7. Rating the quality of evidence – inconsistency. *J Clin Epidemiol* 2011; 64: 1294–1302. doi: 10.1016/j.jclinepi .2011.03.017.
- Guyatt GH, Oxman AD, Kunz R et al. GRADE guidelines: 8. Rating the quality of evidence – indirectness. *J Clin Epidemiol* 2011; 64: 1303–1310. https://doi.org/ 10.1016/j.jclinepi.2011.04.014.
- Guyatt GH, Oxman AD, Sultan S et al. GRADE guidelines: 11. Making an overall rating of confidence in effect estimates for a single outcome and for all outcomes. *J Clin Epidemiol* 2013; 66: 151–157. https://doi.org/10 .1016/j.jclinepi.2012.01.006.
- Hultcrantz M, Rind D, Akl EA et al. The GRADE Working Group clarifies the construct of certainty of evidence. *J Clin Epidemiol* 2017; 87: 4–13.

2. The US Agency for Healthcare Research and Quality (AHRQ) provides a helpful guide for assessing the applicability of interventions to different populations and clinical setting. The term applicability broadly corresponds to the GRADE term directness (usually written as indirectness):

> Atkins D, Chang SM, Gartlehner G et al. Assessing applicability when comparing medical interventions: AHRQ and the effective health care program. *J Clin Epidemiol* 2011; 64: 1198–1207. doi: 10.1016/j.jclinepi.2010.11.021.

Chapter 14: Assessing value

Assessing the value of health care interventions is challenging because of the many issues that need to be assessed and evaluated against each other. The following sources address different components of value.

1. Comparing benefits of treatments with the unintended harms that they may cause is challenging. The following two papers and the work packages of the European Medicines Agency discuss methods of balancing the health gains against the undesirable effects:

   - Pignatti F, Ashby D, Brass EP et al. Structured frameworks to increase the transparency of the assessment of benefits and risks of medicines: current status and possible future directions. *Clin Pharmacol Therap* 2015; 98: 522–533.

   - Kurz, X. Advancing regulatory science, advancing regulatory practice. *Pharmacepidemiol Drug Saf* 2017; 26(6): 722–726. doi: 10.1002/pds.4181.

   - The European Medicines Agency has conducted a series of work packages addressing the methodology of benefit to risk assessment. These have reviewed existing tools and assessed their applicability, tested the utility of new tools, and synthesised a new benefit–risk tool. These can be found on the website: https://www.ema.europa.eu/ en/about-us/support-research/benefit-risk- methodology (accessed 12 October 2021).

2. Several national and international organisations have developed approaches to assessing the value of interventions. The following report and six papers present the methods that have been adopted together with a review of the issues that guided their development:

   - NICE. Guide to the methods of technology appraisal 2013. London: National Institute for Healthcare Excellence. https://www.nice.org.uk/process/pmg9/resources /guide-to-the-methods-of-technology-appraisal -2013-pdf-2007975843781 (accessed 16 January 2021).

- Charlton V. NICE and fair? Health technology assessment policy under the UK's National Institute for Health and Care Excellence, 1999–2018. *Health Care Analysis* 2020; 28: 193–227. https://doi.org/10.1007/s10728-019-00381-x.
- Rehfuess EA, Stratil JM, Scheel IB et al. The WHO-INTEGRATE evidence to decision framework version 1.0: integrating WHO norms and values and a complexity perspective. *BMJ Glob Health* 2019; 4: e000844. doi: 10.1136/bmjgh-2018-000844.
- Stratil JM, Baltussen R, Scheel IB et al. Development of the WHO-INTEGRATE evidence-to-decision framework: an overview of systematic reviews of decision criteria for health decision-making. *Cost Eff Resour Alloc* 2020; 18: 8. https://doi.org/10.1186/s12962-020-0203-6.
- Stratil JM, Paudel D, Setty K et al. Advancing the WHO-INTEGRATE framework as a tool for evidence-informed, deliberative decision-making processes: exploring the views of developers and users of WHO guidelines. The GRADE Evidence to Decision (EtD) framework for health system and public health decisions. *Int J Health Policy Manag* 2020, x(x), 1–13: doi 10.34172/ijhpm.2020.193.
- Baltussen R, Jansen MPM, Bijlmaker L et al. Value assessment frameworks for HTA Agencies: the organization of evidence-informed deliberative processes. *Value Health* 2017; 20: 256–260. doi.org/10.1016/j.jval.2016.11.019.
- Alonso-Ceollo P, Schunemann HJ, Moberg J et al. GRADE Evidence to Decision (EtD) frameworks: a systematic and transparent approach to making well informed healthcare choices. 1: Introduction. *BMJ* 2016; 353: i2016. doi.org/10.1136/bmj.i2016.

3. Multiple criteria decision analysis is a commonly used method for estimating the value of health care interventions. These three papers describe this method:

- Angelis A., Kanavos P. Multiple criteria decision analysis (MCDA) for evaluating new medicines in health technology assessment and beyond: the advance value framework. *Soc Sci Medicine* 2017; 188: 137–156. doi.org/10.1016/j.socscimed.2017.06.024.
- Marsh K, Lanitis T, Neasham D et al. Assessing the value of healthcare interventions using multi-criteria decision analysis: a review of the literature. *PharmacoEconomics* 2014; 32: 345–365. doi: 10.1007/s40273-014-0135-0.
- Jakab I, Nemeth B, Elezbawy B et al. potential criteria for frameworks to support the evaluation of innovative medicines in upper middle-income countries – a systematic literature review on value frameworks and multi-criteria decision analyses. *Frontiers Pharmacol* 2020; 11. doi: 10.3389/fphar.2020.01203.

Index

The Pocket Guide to Critical Appraisal, Second Edition. Iain K. Crombie.
© 2022 John Wiley & Sons Ltd. Published 2022 by John Wiley & Sons Ltd.